A WOMAN'S GUIDE TO MENOPAUSE DOMINATION

MASTER MENOPAUSE WITH CONFIDENCE, FEEL GREAT AND LOOK HOT OVER 50

ELLA RENÉE

CONTENTS

A GIFT TO MY READERS

Please enjoy your own copy of my 10-Day Weight Loss Challenge!

Included in your 10-day challenge is a weight loss meal plan, at home or in the gym exercise program, and daily life-changing habits for long-term weight loss success.

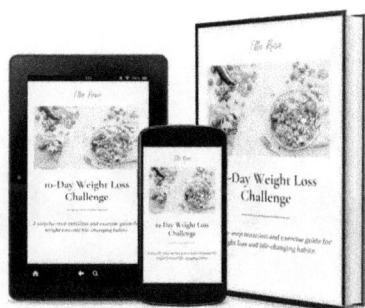

Scan the QR code to download your FREE copy today!

INTRODUCTION

"Women, our bodies change drastically in comparison to men. We're going through menopause. We've got a lot going on and I don't think we've done enough to understand what aging means for women's bodies. What are we supposed to look like? How are we supposed to feel? We are not talking about that enough. The changes, the highs and lows, and the hormonal shifts, there is power in that."

— MICHELLE OBAMA

This is your life on the planet today. You wake up bleary-eyed and force yourself to roll off your bed and head for the bathroom, splash cold water on your face, and get an omelet into your body before heading out for the day. You've been doing this dawn routine for decades now; you don't even need a radio alarm clock anymore to blast you into wakefulness with NPR's *Morning Edition*. You can semi-sleepwalk through the house before drinking your first cup of coffee.

This morning, however, is a bit different. Somehow, you stub your toe on the bathroom door as you try to sidestep your dog, and you suddenly find yourself wide awake, hopping about on one foot until you face a full-length mirror and stop. Who is this tired panda staring back at you with dark circles around her eyes? Is that a tumbleweed on her head? How many furrows does she have on her forehead? Why does she look like she's been left alone in a fully stocked pantry of her favorite foods? You shuffle away quickly, unwilling to confront the truth-telling reflection that has just stared back at you.

Of the many things that can happen to a woman racking up a year each time the Earth circles the sun, menopause is the one that especially tries women's physical, mental, and emotional health to its utmost limits—and no woman is exempt, including you. Not everybody ages as elegantly as Halle Berry or Jane Fonda, so you're one of those left glumly looking at yourself on the shiny metal door of an elevator, wondering where your beach body went and how the beached whale shape has come to take its place.

There's no escaping genetics and the natural order of things, according to scientific studies. Women **are** prone to gaining weight as they grow older, ranging from merely overweight all the way to obesity, and they can point a finger squarely at menopause as the culprit. However, before you start treating this normal life stage like an alien that has hijacked your body for its evil purposes, you must sift through the facts and fiction about it.

Menopause can be a beautiful season in your life, but you're not quite there yet in that perspective because your reality looks like the polar opposite of beauty. Your brain feels packed in wool. You can't remember what you came into the kitchen for, and that scenario plays out several times every day in different rooms of your house. Sleep finds you way past midnight, and you wake up barely two hours later, drenched in sweat. There's also an invisible great wall between your partner and you in bed, which has kept you both from having intimate relations with each other for ages.

Facing the closet has become your new source of dread. You discover items of clothing that no longer fit you when you dress up for the day. Your favorite turtleneck sweater has become a garrote around your neck. With your body parts surrendering to gravity and the inevitable arrival of a slower metabolism, your family's medical history suddenly takes up space in your thoughts. Your dad's hypertension, your mom's diabetes, your aunt's breast cancer—every health issue becomes a little demon in your mind, stirring up irrational fears that rob you of your joy. And all you really want is to be able to feel light enough—literally and figuratively—to run after your grandchildren in their trikes.

It doesn't help that you never seem to have time to take care of yourself. Despite yearly resolutions to do better, you end up eating the fastest meal to order on DoorDash—one full of carbs and fats, which eventually reside in your thighs, upper arms, face, and elsewhere on your body. You do want to live a healthy lifestyle, especially now that menopause is your current companion or soon-to-come aunt with her ill-timed comments over Thanksgiving dinner, but you're like a deer in the headlights, frozen in your tracks and unable to figure out what to do next.

You are not alone in feeling overwhelmed by it all. As time marches on, you become more aware of your mortality, and that can bring about a tsunami of emotions you don't really want to have. One moment, the world assumes a dark and dreary atmosphere, and you want nothing but to curl up into a ball and cry. The next, you want to swing Thor's hammer at your partner's head for no reason at all, although you claim it's because he doesn't help you with the laundry. Even you don't understand where the rage comes from, and it makes you want to go into a tighter fetal position and weep some more.

While it feels like it, it's not the end of the world when menopause comes. You've already taken the first step toward hope by reading this book. This is not the menopause bible, and I'm not a menopause whisperer, but you have the fire in your belly to make things better for yourself. Menopause can be either a monster or a mentor, depending on whether you take the key points here to heart or not. Bottom line is that you want to be in control of your hormones, weight, and everything else affected by menopause. Although there may be some things truly past your abilities and knowledge to manage because Mother Nature says so, you want to be the captain of the ones that can be steered toward a safe haven.

This is not a book of spells to invoke for some abra-cadabra experience. Just like any health and fitness book, it will require you to put in the work (*cue montage of video clips depicting you in beast mode a la boot camp). Even sitting still to finish this book all the way to the last page can take some effort, but it is a good investment of your resources, including time. What you want to come out with from this book are the know-how and skills to be the best you can be, even in the worst throes of menopausal symptoms. It's not a pipe dream to feel comfortable and confident even when the menopause monkey is on your back. You can be and have grace under pressure.

You are experiencing menopause (or are about to) at a time when there are—finally—honest public conversations about it. This is no longer the era when sending girls away to a remote hut for menstruating is acceptable. Or to take them out of school for lack of sanitary napkins. Labeling female bodily functions as a taboo subject or a stigma is no longer de rigueur. What a great time to be alive! Facetiousness aside, this stage of your life comes at no better time when even globally celebrated women have gone on record to discuss their menopausal horrors.

The former US First Lady Michelle Obama was herself hit hard by menopause. She compared her symptoms to having a furnace inside her body and setting it at its highest temperature. Her description evokes an image of flesh and skin sloughing off bones. Oprah was plagued by sleeplessness and heart palpitations, which brings to mind a series of endless nights, tossing and turning for the right pose to welcome—in vain—an absent Morpheus. Gwyneth Paltrow spoke of her emotions running fast and loose like football hooligans in the aftermath of a major match upset. Gillian Anderson shared that she simply felt her life disintegrating without any clear idea as to what was happening to her.

Like rain that drenches mansions and marshes alike, menopause comes to all women, regardless of socioeconomic status, educational background, or choice between tea and coffee. When you know that it's inescapable, you are left with a decision to make: to embrace it and make some proverbial lemonade from the situation or to fight it as furiously as the men of Rohan and the Elves fought the Orcs in the Battle of Helm's Deep. This being the 21st century, I imagine you're one of those people who already have full plates to deal with every day. Menopause shouldn't be another item to add on to yours. Even if you have no choice, it shouldn't be the entrée.

I'm still a few years away from my own menopause, but I have spent almost 20 years of my life in the health and fitness industry, where menopause is an oft-discussed topic. It has its own mile marker on the highway of every woman's narrative. Even men can't help but notice it because their relationships with the women in their lives also change. Kids can sense something is up as their moms, aunts, and grandmas start behaving and looking differently.

Within my space, I have met many women who have sought advice on diets for balancing their hormones and other necessary lifestyle changes to confront menopause with a brave face. I have happily done this for them because of my background in nutritional science. Over the years, that knowledge has grown significantly as I research, discuss with, and learn first-hand from experts. I have been the shoulder to cry on for many women struggling through insane hormonal changes. I have coached them on how to prioritize their health and fitness in order to come out whole on the other side. In a nutshell, menopause is no stranger to me.

When you and I take a journey together in this book, I'm holding your hand as I have done for other women who have come before you. Their stories motivated me to write this and approach menopause from a different tangent. I'm just really here to help you, and them discover ways of experiencing menopause on your own terms. Your menopause is your own; if you decide to possess it, you gain power over it. I'm determined to assist you in feeling confident about yourself as you navigate the minefield. This is no time to be afraid or worried. There are safe routes out of it, and I'm here to shine a light down the paths from which you can choose. More than anything else, I wrote this book because I want other women to wield the knowledge and information that can put menopause in its proper perspective. If, at the end of reading this book, you can embrace your menopause as a special season of your life, then I would have done my job. I would want for you to manage your symptoms, lose weight, and fall in love with your body and yourself (again).

Remember that there isn't a quick fix anywhere in the pages of this book for weathering menopause. Numerous women have done nothing but vent their frustrations at trying out a whole plethora of formulas, dos and don'ts, exercises, diets, etc., to no avail. Instead, I offer you a principle or set of principles that can guide you through menopause and its attendant issues, regardless of the nuances and idiosyncrasies of your situation. It caters to your unique circumstances so you can be quick on your feet to adapt to the curveballs that menopause can throw at you. This is your chance to read about them and learn them. While this book can't help you prevent menopause from ever coming your way, it can equip you well enough to dominate your menopause.

1

MENOPAUSE UNLEASHED: WHAT'S HAPPENING TO MY BODY?

B ack in the early 2000s, a British comedy film came out about a group of older women who organize and execute an annual calendar for their women's society. While it all sounds so tame and full of goodwill in the spirit of fundraising, the punchline comes when the audience realizes that all these dignified church women were going to pose in the nude, one for each month of the year and all together for a December spread.

Hilarity ensues, of course, but more than the belly laughs, *Calendar Girls* reminds everyone that there is beauty even in the golden years of one's life—saggy breasts, triple chins, leathery skins, and all. Even the exquisite Helen Mirren shows the viewers that none of that matters as she romps around onscreen with her chest bare for all to see. The point of the older-chick flick is that the graying heads of flawed but evolving women are as lovely to behold as those of youthful beauty pageant contestants. What matters in the end is their friendships, children, partners, and greasy fries after an easygoing yoga session up a breezy hill.

Since the movie is based on a true story, you can conclude that there truly are women out there who have ridden the wave of menopause triumphantly without falling off the surfboard and hitting their heads on a coral reef. They live among us, exuding attractiveness inside and out. When it comes to you, however, you have serious doubts about your chances of survival. You've seen how it was with your mom or your aunt or your university professor before and how each transformed into a grumpy old woman. Your deepest fear is that you have the same Ms. Hyde, hiding somewhere in the recesses of your persona, waiting to give you a nasty surprise in the middle of menopause. Can your partner withstand such a visitation from your inner grump? How about your children? Your colleagues? Your friends?

While you have reason to worry about how you may turn out to be in menopause, you can come prepared for the showdown. As always, preparation begins with arming yourself with enough knowledge about it. It's not sufficient to think of menopause as the time when your menstruation comes to a full stop. It's not simply the season when you say goodbye to the period products aisle of the supermarket. This is the superficial information about menopause, but there is so much more about this bodily transformation to know.

WHAT'S MENOPAUSE AND WHY IS MY BODY THROWING A TANTRUM?

While younger women can miss their periods because of pregnancy, stress, or underlying health issues, to name a few, the truly menopausal women are the ones who miss theirs every month for at least a whole year. This may come as a welcome cessation for women who couldn't be bothered by tampons and dreams of their own flesh-and-blood children, but it can be devastating news for those who still hold out for hope of their own babies.

From Nature's perspective, it's possible to view the arrival of menopause in your 40s or 50s as a long enough delay of the inevitable. "Okay, ma'am. Menopause really has to board the bus now. It's waited four decades to join you on your journey." Whether you like it or not, that bus door has got to swing open to let it in. And you need to allow it because it's a legit, ticketed passenger.

On average, menopause begins at age 51, although period termination can happen anytime between 45 to 55 years old. Some women's ovaries can begin to decline way before the said age range, while others can continue to menstruate way into the higher 50s. Menopause can make an early entrance if you've never given birth to a baby. In contrast, it can be delayed if you've had at least one pregnancy. There's no one-size-fits-all rule for menopause's arrival and duration because it may be determined by genetics. If the women in your family had an early menopause, there is a possibility that you will as well, but there are no guarantees on that. Lifestyle nitty-gritty (for example, smoking) and health situations (for example, cancer treatment protocols) can also affect your experience of menopause. Smoking is actually known to be a cause of the early-bird menopause. The bottom line is that menopause is going to be very different from one woman to the next.

It's possible that menopause can come upon you without you knowing it, especially if you've had your uterus removed in a hysterectomy. The same is true if you've had an endometrial ablation, which is the removal of your uterine lining, a treatment for anyone with heavy periods. You can remain blissfully unaware until hot flashes descend upon your peaceful existence, after which your life will never be the same again. If none of the usual symptoms manifests themselves in your body, a blood test can also reveal your estrogen level, a key indicator of the presence or absence of menopause.

STAGES OF MENOPAUSE – FROM MILDLY CONFUSED TO FULL-ON HOT MESS

Menopause signals the start of changes to your body to prepare you for—well—old age or—if you want to sprinkle fairy dust on it—the golden years. You certainly can't keep popping out babies way into your late 90s for many obvious, common-sensical reasons. That's why estrogen and progesterone hormones must begin decreasing production as you move closer to the half-century mark of your life.

Just before menopause, there's a period known as peri-menopause, when your body starts to transition. Hormones begin their inexorable drop. Some menopausal symptoms start making a cameo appearance. Your periods no longer come like clockwork. The interval between your periods can become either longer or shorter. You might skip a month or two entirely before it makes another appearance. The amount of blood you expel can go higher or lower than normal, so you can never know if you have enough tampons or pads on hand. The 'fun' part is that you may bleed between periods, so pantyliners may be necessary to include in your next shopping run.

Hot flashes become a reality in your world as peri-menopause begins. However, for as long as you still have a menstrual cycle within a 12-month stretch, you're not quite into full-on menopause yet. Perimenopause can take anywhere from two to eight years before menopause finally plants itself firmly in your body. Until it does, expect to have your menstruation stop and start and stop again in a random pattern. You can think of perimenopause as a rehearsal leading to the real thing.

Despite the irregular periods in perimenopause, you can still get pregnant. This is important to remember if you're not planning to have kids. If you're on a birth control method, you should continue applying it, especially since ovulation becomes unpredictable. Not until menopause is fully upon you can you safely stop. However, don't forget that some birth control methods are more than a barrier to pregnancy. They are also a means of protecting you from sexually transmitted infections or diseases.

With the lowering of your hormone production, you experience a surplus of new goings-on in your body. One of the most discussed is hot flashes. It would be nice to think of it as a superpower similar to the Flash's ability to move at hyper speed, but it's not a phenomenon measurable by a speedometer. Try a thermometer instead because hot flashes are a feeling of extreme heat emanating from inside your body. Only you can sense it, which can be very frustrating. How can you explain to your partner just how uncomfortable you are with their arms wrapped around your body while you sweat waterfalls in silence? Your skin gets all flush, you have tingles at your fingertips, and your heart races as though you were chasing after an ice cream truck in your childhood. Without a moment's rest, cold chills can take over a hot flash, and you're still in the same bind of wanting to crawl out of your skin.

Hot flashes can happen at any time. Former US First Lady Michelle Obama's significant experience of it was on board Marine One, a helicopter designated exclusively for the US president's use, surely on the way to some event or another. If that happened to you in full view of the public eye, you'd certainly feel properly mortified and ready to crawl under a large boulder. No woman has the power to stop a hot flash from occurring. However, I will provide you with the knowledge on how to minimize your symptoms and save you from an embarrassing situation.

Another common symptom of menopause is weight gain. Your decreased estrogen supply causes your metabolism to slow down significantly. You can no longer eat as greedily as a Great Dane because your body is losing its ability to convert all those calories to expendable energy. Your less-active lifestyle—blame it all on thee busyness of work and other adulting responsibilities that take you away from the gym— compounds the issue because you cut off any chance for your body to burn carbs and fats. You might even accuse your slothful metabolism of making you disinclined to exercise and other physical activities.

To top things off, it's like the universe decided to put on its director's hat and said, "You know what would be a real knee-slapper? Vaginal dryness!" Menopause causes the physiology of your vagina to change. As your estrogen levels go down, your vaginal tissues begin to thin out and/or inflame, making sexual intercourse a rather unpleasant experience. This vaginal atrophy leads to vaginal dryness, compounding your discomfort but making personal lube manufacturers go ka-ching at cash registers whenever you and your partner plan a "Netflix and chill" night.

With estrogen's grand exit, inflammation can become the life of the party. It's like inviting a group of rowdy teenagers to a library – things get a little chaotic. Suddenly, your bones and joints are throwing a party of their own, complete with surprise aches and pains. But fear not because there is hope that comes in the form of strengthening exercises!

Menopause doesn't just affect the physical but the mental and emotional as well; be ready to cope with crazy mood swings. You can find yourself in either a deep funk or an irrational rage at any given moment. Nothing that you feel aligns with actual circumstances, leaving you baffled by everything. You can be in the middle of your own birthday party, but you have Eeyore on your back, and you don't feel very festive about the whole thing. It's a default move to blame everything on your fluctuating hormones, but that's just a shorthand explanation. Other factors like your evolving circumstances or the basic fact of aging, which even men experience, can come into play to influence your emotions. Regardless of the specific trigger, your pendulum-like emotions will affect the people around you, so you need to help them expect the unexpected from you.

Insomnia can also plague you in menopause, although this may not be an obvious sign to you if you've always had problems sleeping. Tossing and turning in bed will be an understated description of your experience. With hot flashes thrown into the mix, your sleeping problems can feel like an attack of invisible aliens on your body and sanity. It's never a pleasant experience to lie in bed and stare at your ceiling for hours on end, with an occasional mosquito or shifting shadow to break the monotony.

If insomnia isn't already knocking your brain off its pedestal from lack of rest and sleep, trust that menopause itself will certainly compromise the quality of your thoughts. And it's not just going to be the whole "where the heck are my keys" syndrome either. You'll start forgetting simple words, so "whatchamacallit" and "thingamajig" become your all-purpose terms for the ones you can't remember. Even the name of your neighbor of 20 years falls into the brain fog zone, and you berate yourself for being such an awful fellow resident.

After menopause comes postmenopause. Once menopause takes up full-time and permanent residence in your body, that's it. You can no longer have a period every month or get pregnant. You have to be some sort of unicorn to have a resumption of menstruation after menopause. That rarely ever happens, especially if you've not had the monthly visitor in well over two years. If in case it does return, you must see your doctor immediately because it might indicate a serious condition that's only now blipping on your radar.

Postmenopause can begin two to five years after your last period. By then, you can bid a fond and final farewell to all the symptoms that plagued you at the height of your menopausal years. I'm very certain that you won't miss your hot flashes, although they might still make a comeback years later just to poke your inner bear. Don't worry though, they're unlikely to overstay like every Airbnb host's worst nightmare.

ARE MY OVARIES RETIRING? TESTING FOR MENOPAUSE

While all these signs and symptoms of menopause are enough to send you running for the hills, they shouldn't be made to take over your entire life. Simple preparedness is often all you need to keep you standing firmly in place. One way of getting ready is knowing exactly how things stand with your body. Have yourself tested for your FSH and estrogen levels. The letters stand for follicle-stimulating hormone, which your pituitary gland produces. The amount of FSH you have determines where you're at in your sexual development and function timeline. This particular test shouldn't be expensive since there are over-the-counter test kits you can conduct on yourself from the comfort of your home—science and technology have come a long way, baby!

FSH is responsible for stimulating egg maturation and producing estradiol. Estradiol is estrogen with a specific task: to regulate periods and support women's reproductive tract. When you measure your FSH, you determine not only your hormone levels but also the presence of some pituitary conditions.

One test introduced in the past few years measures the amount of anti-Mullerian hormone in your blood. One important thing you learn from knowing your AMH level is the number of potential egg cells you have left. This is vital data for any woman still hoping for her own baby. Otherwise, that information tells your doctor when you should expect menopause to come knocking on your door, if it hasn't done so yet.

I mentioned home tests earlier, and here are my insights about them. Home kits are very convenient and rob you of any excuse for not doing the test, but there may be cases when you simply must see a physician, especially when your symptoms are just way too extraordinary to be overlooked. There are other bodily issues that can masquerade as menopause, so you want to rule those ones out before issuing a press release on how special you are. The doctor may want to exclude thyroid problems because hypothyroidism (minimal activity of the thyroid, causing changes in the metabolism) is its own disorder and requires a different set of treatment protocols. You may be prescribed one that verifies your TSH level to check thyroid function.

Your doctor might also suggest a pregnancy test, which can be another reason for your body acting up.

The important thing in taking a test or battery of tests is knowing and dealing with the actual issue. It will be very frustrating for you to spend so much on one treatment when you actually need a different one. That's like an example of very bad medical dark humor: amputating the right leg when it was the left that had to be removed.

Home tests are more than just convenient; they are suitable especially for women who have hot flashes, irregular menstruation, and vaginal dryness at an unusual time, say, much too early for the symptoms to appear. Once you can eliminate these experiences as being related to menopause, you should find out other possible causes for your own good health and peace of mind. None of these symptoms is pleasant, so the sooner you can figure out what's going on with your body, the better for your overall well-being.

Home tests are convenient because they're readily available at a pharmacy down the road or online, but they may not be definitive enough to tell you if you're in menopause or perimenopause. What they do provide is sufficient info for you to process so you can decide whether or not to seek further consultation with a health professional. Part of the convenience is also based on the speed by which you can get your results. Some tests guarantee a turnaround of a mere few days; others may take a week to get back to you. How much patience can you exercise to wait for results?

The method of sample collection is also very important to consider when buying a test kit. While some tests require just saliva, others need for you to prick your finger. The saliva method isn't as accurate as the finger prick one, which necessitates the drawing of your blood, but it may be your saving grace if you're deathly afraid of needles.

Another thing to consider when buying a home test is certification. This is one of those moments when you must be a bit obsessive-compulsive and read the label on the product box. You want a test that goes straight to a lab with CLIA certification for processing. CLIA stands for Clinical Laboratory Improvement Amendments, so a CLIA-certified lab is one that adheres to federal standards for testing human specimens. It is inspected regularly to maintain its certification so that you can rest easy about your specimen accidentally mixing up with an inbound virus-infected tourist. You can trust the results from such a lab to assess your health and reveal any issue that may need further investigation.

You may note from reading different tests' fine print that some of them offer free doctor consults, regardless of the results. That's more bang for your buck, especially if you want to be fully ready for menopause. If you can find one that offers such, you must definitely take it or at least give it some serious thought. Healthcare can become quite expensive in the long term, especially in the United States of America. Every bit of savings or freebies should be exploited. A single kit can cost more than a dozen and a half coffee Trenta at Starbucks in December; make sure you get one that gives you the value you want, or you may seriously regret missing out on that cold caffeine fix.

BUSTING MENOPAUSE MYTHS

Once you've firmly established that you're in perimenopause, menopause, or postmenopause, you may want to brace yourself instinctively for the rough ride ahead. I don't blame you. Majority of what you hear out there sounds like the writings of Anne Rice and Stephen King combined, filling you with dread. However, you need to separate fact from fiction if you are to survive the season. Truth does set you free, even if it isn't always pleasant to hear.

One important myth to bust is the horrible experience you get when menopause hits you. While all the symptoms I've described here are true and can be quite challenging to deal with, depending on your adaptability to change, they are not going to hound you 24/7 for the entire season of a few or several years. Hot flashes can come suddenly and knock you down for a bit, but you won't stay down from them for the rest of your life. Your weight gain may suck, but it's not what's going to define you, and it's most certainly not a permanent fixture of your body. You may even end up living through menopause without noticing it because all your symptoms are a timid lot. They enter and exit without making a sound. One or two symptoms may sometimes jolt you into a panic (your brain fog causes you to forget the name of your aunt who babysat you for many years), but the intensity of that panic fades away. Your periods may stop and start like a stick-shift car in the hands of a student driver, but they eventually go away for good. A time will come when you won't even remember what it was like to have them. Your attitude toward and approach to menopause will have a whole lot to do with how menopause is going to look in your life. In other words, it doesn't have to be an awful time for you.

Another myth to debunk is that menopause is your personal Pennywise and something to be feared. How could you be afraid of something that's part of your maturing process as a human being? Yes, menopause signals change, but the change it brings is similar to what a caterpillar undergoes as it becomes a butterfly. It's a beautiful metamorphosis when your body ceases to function in a certain way so you can be free to explore new interests and focus on different experiences.

The knee-jerk reaction to "change" and "difference" is to run in the opposite direction, but this book can show you an alternative way of dealing with them. As I'm writing this part, I remember Heimlich, the caterpillar in Pixar's *A Bug's Life*, who was always excited by the prospect of one day becoming a butterfly. He talked about it endlessly to anyone who dared give him an audience. That's the appropriate and ideal reaction we should have when welcoming menopause into our lives. The transformation it brings can be harnessed for good.

A third myth to throw away is that you're menopausal once your period stops. There's a reason why there's a stage called perimenopausal. You begin to experience the symptoms, but they're not quite full-blown yet. Think of them as the entourage in a royal procession. They all bear the same pomp and circumstance as the monarch to demand your attention, but they can never be the monarch. The cessation of your period is just your body announcing the arrival of something important; it's not the main attraction. And as I've established earlier, your period has to be missing in action for at least 12 months before you can claim and play the menopause card.

While a majority of the talk surrounding menopause pegs it as a rather tragic occurrence, it really isn't. It doesn't have to be. That's just another myth to tear down. Instead of focusing on the difficulties it brings, start zeroing in on the pluses. You won't ever experience premenstrual syndrome again. Goodbye, binge eating! Goodbye, knee-buckling stomach cramps! Goodbye, headache for days! All that is going to be behind you now.

You don't have to worry anymore about bleeding in the middle of a movie with no period products available on hand. Your bedsheets and underwear don't become canvases of crimson leaks. You no longer concern yourself with surprise pregnancies. You can finally throw away your IUD and pills—just don't stop using condoms and other similar prophylaxes if you play the field to protect yourself from STIs. As you can see from all these examples, menopause isn't all doom and gloom. If you keep yourself in top form, there are still plenty of years ahead of you.

Menopause doesn't automatically mean that you're old. While it does happen in your latter years, the numbers don't really mean anything in the long run. There are plenty of menopausal women out there who do downward dogs better than I can. They still ride their mountain bikes every weekend down a forest trail. They can run as fast as their grandchildren around the park. "Old" is a concept that means something different to different people. Don't forget that menopause can happen even in your 30s or 40s, depending on your general well-being. Cancer, for instance, can cause your menses to stop at a much earlier age, so menopause can never pass as an age gauge.

One myth about menopause worth busting is that weight gain is automatic and happens to all. While misery loves company and wants you to hang on to that myth, the truth is that it's neither automatic nor every woman's experience. With a lifestyle of healthy eating and living, you stand to avoid the whole weight gain pitfall of menopause.

Even as your metabolism slows down because estrogen has decided to leave the building, your hormone production actually continues to run as before. What your body does in menopause is that it reworks the hierarchy of hormone production. Some hormones, similar or related to estrogen, decline in quantities produced, while others increase. Others simply have to be retired because, for example, your childbearing abilities have to be curtailed past a certain age for your own safety and the baby's.

By now, you should be fully aware that hot flashes aren't the only symptoms of menopause. Believing this myth doesn't prepare you well for the breadth and depth of bodily change. Menopause is 3D; focusing on just hot flashes makes the whole thing flat in 2D. You must account for brain fog, night sweats, insomnia, and other symptoms. It's not that you must know all of them so you can "treat" menopause. On the contrary, thinking that you can or can't treat menopause is completely fake news.

Menopause isn't a disease that requires (or doesn't require) treatment. It's one of your body's natural processes. That doesn't mean you can't find ways to alleviate its symptoms because you can—just don't treat it like an invasion of body snatchers. It's as much a part of you as your skin, your smile, and the soles of your feet. You have to learn to cherish it as a valuable season of your life, an important milestone down your own highway.

Stephanie's Story

When Stephanie hit her early 50s, her menopausal symptoms arrived like clockwork—such has always been her experience since puberty when it came to her reproductive functions. Since Stephanie wasn't blind-sided by the whole thing, she met their onset with open arms and celebrated her bodily transformation with a ceremonial handover of her stockpile of period products to her daughter, who wasn't too thrilled to use her mom's old—and possibly expired—stuff.

Despite her daughter's lack of enthusiasm for the free-bies, Stephanie was ecstatic. She felt like a woman unshackled from all those modern-day female aids. Without her period to cramp her style, she could finally plan holidays that involved feeding her "wild side," that is, her sense of adventure into the bush. She didn't care if the camping grounds she planned to stay at had no plumbing or electricity. She began looking at safaris to different African countries while checking out the online REI Shop.

Every so often in her planning, Stephanie had to pause for a bit as wave upon wave of hot flashes sent her into a state of vertigo and confusion. She knew to expect them, so she bore all of them quietly—the same with the headaches, blurry vision, and night sweats. She tried to avoid other people during these bouts, knowing she was not the best company during these times. There were new symptoms coming in, though, that she felt needed a physician consult. Even when she was quite excited about her upcoming holiday plans, something at the back of her mind bugged her and made her feel that she was too old for such an adventure. It was turning her smile upside down, so she needed to check in with someone who could diagnose her mental and emotional states correctly. If it were menopause-related depression, at least she could equip herself with the right tools, knowledge, and maybe drugs to counteract the worst of it. It felt good to be in a position to view menopause in a matter-of-fact way. She wasn't going to repeat her mom's experience of being an out-of-control wrecking ball.

While you may see a lot of physical manifestations of menopause in yourself and other women, the majority of what's really going on during the season happens in the background or in unseen places because that's where your hormones stay. In the next chapter, you get to delve deeper into the hidden world of your hormones and how these invisible components of your body chemistry command the room and dictate much of what happens to your body as it matures.

2

WHAT'S WITH THE HORMONES?

Once your body decides it no longer wants you to have kids, it begins to change the way your hormones work. Quite frankly, it should be illegal that our bodies do not ask for permission first. I mean, after 30-40 years of periods, we *finally* get used to the hormonal ups and downs of a menstrual cycle, only for our bodies to decide it needs to change once again. What a diva!

Estrogen and progesterone are the two most important hormones in a woman's body. If your hormones were in high school, estrogen and progesterone would be the popular girls that got invited to all the parties. In fact, as most scientists would tell you, they are the cool hormones invited to all the parties. They affect so many functions of your body that it's quite ironic how much we take them for granted on a day-to-day basis. That's exactly why perimenopause and menopause are such a challenging transformation for women. The popular girls who made life feel like a warm burst of sunshine are suddenly no longer bubbly. They rarely make an appearance, and when they do, they don't seem as full of life anymore!

With the popular girls gone, you start to experience a natural decline in estrogen and progesterone hormones. This then leads to common menopause symptoms like hot flashes, vaginal dryness, and weight gain.

In this chapter, we will be acting as menopause detectives, investigating what happened to estrogen, progesterone, and all the other cool girls in your body and why they have suddenly stopped showing up to parties! Or, to be more scientific, we'll examine how hormonal imbalance triggers menopause.

WHY ARE MY HORMONES THROWING A FRAT PARTY?

Menopause is quite similar to puberty in that it radically changes your hormonal balance. In the case of puberty, this change happens to prepare you for your fertile (reproductive) years, while in the case of menopause, it occurs to prepare you for your post-menopausal years.

Estrogen and progesterone are produced in our ovaries. As women, our ovaries are very important body parts. It is weird to think about since we generally can't see our ovaries. However, it solidifies itself as the boss since it produces these two popular girl hormones.

We keep talking about hormone-this, hormone-that, but if you don't understand too clearly what hormones are, you may actually be confused. Well, hormones are pretty much just chemical messengers that travel to different parts of your body to deliver a command. They travel through your bloodstream, using it as a passageway to send messages to your organs and tissues. These messages/commands control very important body functions, from hunger to satiety, ovulation to menstruation, sleepiness to alertness, happiness to depression, and just a general sense of balance in all parts of your body (known as homeostasis).

Hormones are created in your endocrine system. The endocrine system is a collection of organs in your body known as glands. If your glands were a management firm, then your ovaries would be mid-management, while your pituitary glands would be the CEO. Dr. Divya Yogi-Morren, an endocrinologist (i.e., a hormone doctor), explains pituitary glands as the glands "responsible for making hormones that tell the other glands what hormones they should make." Your pituitary gland, despite being a CEO, is a small pea-sized gland that lives in your hypothalamus, which is a fancy way of saying "the base of your brain."

In general, if everything is in a good balance, you achieve hormonal balance: you have the right amount of all the different types of hormones in your body. When you have hormonal imbalance, on the other hand, you have too little or too much of one or more hormones. (This is where your hormones call everyone to the frat party). You may think of hormones as just chemicals, but these chemical signals are so important that just a little imbalance can lead to serious and/or life-altering conditions. Cough, cough, menopause!

During menopause, your body is essentially trying to find a new normal: a new hormonal balance for your post-reproductive years. While it is going through this process, your hormones are imbalanced, leading to the annoying symptoms. Some women are lucky, and their body eventually finds a balance. Other women are not so lucky postmenopause and stay imbalanced. If this happens to you, you don't need to worry. Thanks to advances in modern science, there are ways to try to correct or make up for this imbalance, whether through medicine or lifestyle, as we will discuss later in this chapter.

So far, scientists have identified more than fifty hormones in our bodies. As important as they are, unless you are a scientist, let's be honest, we just don't care that much to learn about fifty different hormones and their purposes. In the previous chapter, you already became acquainted with estrogen, progesterone, and FSH. They make part of the *Squad of Seven*, the seven boss hormones that are considered the really important ones. The other four are cortisol (the hormone your body releases when you are stressed), testosterone (a male sex hormone that both men and women produce), thyroid (which controls your body's metabolism), and growth hormone (which does what it says on the tin and is responsible for our physical growth as children and teenagers). Other important hormones that affect or are affected by menopause are anti-Mullerian hormone (AMH) and Luteinizing Hormone (LH), which play a vital part in the development of our bodies.

Now we know the basics we need to know about hormones, let's dig a little deeper. We know that menopause is a result of hormonal imbalance, and your body struggles to find homeostasis because of sudden hormonal changes. But what does that really mean?

HORMONES AFFECTED BY MENOPAUSE

You can't talk about menopause without talking about eggs. No, not supermarket eggs. Women typically don't lay shelled eggs. If you do, you might want to see a doctor.

Our female bodies are pretty spectacular once you get down to the nitty-gritty of how it works! Essentially, we are born with all the eggs we will ever have. That's right! When you arrive in this world as a newborn, you arrive with a packed suitcase filled with a lifetime supply of eggs. This suitcase is technically known as your follicles, which are located in your ovaries. Then your body waits. Once it judges you can now carry a child (or it gets too impatient, as in the case of very young girls who get their first period before they even turn ten), it slaps you with puberty and begins releasing eggs. Your menstrual cycle begins. It's quite spectacular to think that the eggs that would ultimately become your children were in you even while your own mother was carrying you as a fetus! Nature is pretty impressive when she wants to be.

As fetuses in our mother's womb, we have about 6 million eggs. Nature doesn't want to take chances and is desperate for you to reproduce, so she overpacks. By the time we are born this decreases to 1 million eggs.

By the time you reach puberty, the number of eggs has now decreased to 300,000 eggs. By the time you reach menopause, you only have about 1,000 eggs left and they are usually not the best quality either. Nature decides it is time you retire from reproducing.

Once it notices that you no longer have many eggs, your ovaries throw in the towel. After working non-stop for the past three to five decades, your ovaries just want to sit back, read a John Grisham novel and sip a relaxing chamomile tea. So, when Luteinizing Hormone (LH) and Follicle-Stimulating Hormone (FSH) (both of which are made in your pituitary gland) send them a message, they leave it on read most of the time. It's kind of rude to be honest. Your ovaries also begin to produce fewer hormones, namely estrogen and progesterone. Since your retired ovaries are now releasing fewer hormones, LH and FSH now find it difficult to do their job because their boss is not backing them up. They can't regulate estrogen, progesterone, and testosterone on their own, so your body responds to this by settling into menopause.

Hence, you can now say that you know the root cause of menopause: your ovaries retire! This causes hormonal imbalance, particularly the balance of the big shot hormones: estrogen, progesterone, and testosterone.

Estrogen

Estrogen is very much a feminine hormone. During puberty, estrogen causes bodily changes and the development of what is known as secondary sex characteristics, such as your breasts and hips. She's essentially one of nature's employees (or pimps), trying very hard to get you pregnant. It's part of nature's weird obsession with causing you to reproduce.

A sex and reproductive hormone, estrogen is responsible for your menstrual cycle, ovulation, pregnancy, and menopause. There are three types of estrogen:

- Estrone (E1)

This is a weak estrogen. It is the main estrogen that your body makes following menopause.

- Estradiol (E2)

This is a strong form of estrogen. It is the main estrogen your body makes during your fertile (reproductive) years. She is the head pimp trying to get you pregnant.

- Estriol (E3)

Another weak estrogen, estriol, is the type of estrogen that your body produces during pregnancy. It keeps your uterus healthy and prepares your body for childbirth and breastfeeding.

Estrogen is responsible for more than sexual and reproductive processes in your body. It is also a key player in your cardiovascular system (helping to maintain healthy cholesterol levels), your skeletal system (influencing how your body uses the mineral calcium and maintains strong bones), your central nervous system, and even maintaining the health of your vagina. Indeed, estrogen plays a key role in your:

- Blood flow and circulation
- Muscle mass
- Bone health
- Cholesterol levels
- Blood glucose levels
- Skin moisture and collagen production
- Brain function

This hormone is made mostly in your ovaries. However, small doses are also produced in your adrenal glands (which is located at the top of your kidneys) and your adipose tissue (which is your body fat).

Once you enter perimenopause, your ovaries tap out. Your estrogen levels begin to seriously drop. By the time you enter menopause, your main form of estrogen changes from estradiol to estrone. You will be able to tell you have low estrogen levels from these symptoms:

- Trouble concentrating
- Dry skin
- Moodiness or irritability
- Weight gain, particularly around the abdomen
- Vaginal dryness
- Weak, brittle bones
- Headaches
- Hot flashes
- Night sweats
- Irregular periods or no periods
- Painful intercourse
- Decreased sex drive
- Fatigue
- Difficulty sleeping

Progesterone

Progesterone, like estrogen, supports pregnancy and menstruation. It is typically known as the pregnancy hormone, preparing your uterus for the arrival of a fertilized egg and also maintaining pregnancies to term.

Nature might be a pimp, but she takes care of her girls when they finally do reproduce!

Progesterone also has other functions, such as regulating your blood pressure and improving your mood and sleep.

Once it is no longer needed during perimenopause, progesterone levels drop. You will be able to tell you have low progesterone levels from these symptoms:

- Changes in your mood
- Loss of bone density
- Irregular menstruation cycle and bleeding
- Migraines and headaches

Testosterone

Another sex hormone, testosterone, is produced in your ovaries. Most of it is converted into estradiol. The rest is used to increase libido, muscle mass, and control fat distribution.

Since testosterone levels naturally drop with increased age in both women and men, your testosterone levels fall even lower during perimenopause and menopause.

You will be able to tell you have low testosterone level from these symptoms:

- Irregular menstrual cycles
- Decreased sex drive and sexual satisfaction
- Weight gain
- Fatigue and sluggishness
- Muscle weakness
- Vaginal dryness
- Fertility issues
- Loss of bone density
- Sleep disturbances

Although your ovaries stop producing estrogen during menopause, the story does not end there. They may have retired, but they still make pot holders as a hobby - pot holders that they sell at their local farmer's market on the weekends. In this case, the pot holders are small amounts of testosterone, which is then converted into estradiol.

Your adrenal glands are also still working. They continue to produce a hormone known as androstenedione, which is then converted into estrone and estradiol. So, while the boss may have retired, your body finds a replacement to cover her: your adrenal glands. Nonetheless, this replacement only covers her most basic responsibilities, and your body is producing far less estrogen (both in quantity and strength) than it used to during your reproductive years. Nature has decided you just don't need it anymore. And if this causes a painful transition for you, you can leave a message with nature and she'll get back to you when Hell freezes over!

Alternatively, you can buckle up, decide you won't let nature win, and learn how to live a happy life during and following menopause. Hint: Most women choose the latter!

The Effects of Menopause on the Body

Since menopause affects your hormones, it is only natural that this then affects your different bodily systems. Why? Well, these systems are now receiving little or no messages, unlike before when your ovaries were heavily involved in the process. The following systems are particularly affected by menopause:

• The endocrine system

Your endocrine system is a system of hormones and glands that controls your reproduction, growth, and metabolism. Menopause affects your endocrine system, causing:

- Hot flashes
- Weight gain, particularly in your abdomen
- Stopping your menstrual cycle

- **The nervous system**

Your nervous system is also powered, controlled, and influenced by your hormones. Menopause affects your nervous system, causing:

- Rapid mood swings
- Anxiety
- Depression-like feelings
- Sleep problems
- Hot flashes
- Night sweats
- Memory problems

- **Cardiovascular system**

Lower levels of estrogen may affect your cardiovascular system, increasing your risk of developing cardiovascular disease. Since low estrogen levels also play a part in increasing cholesterol levels, this also increases your chance of a heart attack or stroke.

- **Immune and excretory systems**

Once again, estrogen levels cause a difference in how these systems function. Low estrogen levels sometimes lead to incontinence, i.e., your bladder leaking uncontrollably during your daily life activities. Low estrogen levels also cause frequent urination. This may prompt you to get up at night more often, causing sleep disturbances and, as a result, bad health.

• **Skeletal and muscular system**

Bone density loss is commonly caused by menopause (as we've discussed above). This is a leading cause of osteoporosis and bone fractures in women.

Menopause also often causes the loss of muscle mass as well as stiff and achy joints.

TAMING THE HORMONE HURRICANE: HOW TO TREAT HORMONAL CHANGES DURING MENOPAUSE

You left a few messages for Nature and she still hasn't gotten back to you. You're beginning to think she never will. Life has to go on somehow. The only solution might be to turn to science since your ex-pimp is shirking responsibility. Good old science! She's responsible! She'll take care of you!

The effects of menopause on the body are not exactly something to throw a parade over. If only menopause brought with it super intelligence and beautiful supple skin, then women wouldn't even complain! In fact, there would be a black market drug to induce menopause earlier, so we can all look like juicy, healthy goddesses!

Many of my clients have confided in me that the early stages of menopause were quite challenging for them not only because they had to learn how to live with unpleasant symptoms, but also because it felt like they had to learn how to live in their bodies all over again. You are dealing not only with the physical changes, but also with the emotional and mental challenges that come with that.

It's daunting the first time you think about it, but once you familiarize yourself with the treatment options available to you, a lot of that negativity will seep away. Life will seem much breezier. Butterflies will seem more alive and filled with color, and your hot flashes won't seem to bother just as much. Where, before, you used to call your ex-pimp incessantly, desperate for her to return, you can finally let her go. Pssh! You don't need her! You're a survivor and an independent woman!

Hormonal Therapies

Since menopause is a hormone-based change, hormone therapy (HT) is sometimes used to bring back a sense of balance to your body. Hormones are very delicate, so doctors don't like to recommend hormone therapy unless you meet certain specifications. In addition, it does come with risks - like most medications and more research needs to be done since it is a relatively new treatment option.

Hormone therapy increases your estrogen and/or progesterone levels. By doing so, it works to alleviate and minimize menopausal symptoms. If you feel you will benefit from hormone therapy, talk to your doctor about it. Your doctor will examine factors such as your age, personal medical history, family's medical history and the types and severity of menopause symptoms you have to determine if hormone therapy is right for you. There are two types of hormone therapy:

1. Estrogen therapy

This involves taking a pill, using a patch, using a vaginal ring, gel or spray or using a cream containing a low dose of estrogen.

2. Estrogen Progesterone/Progestin Hormone Therapy (EPT)

This combines both progesterone and estrogen therapy together. In some cases, progesterone is replaced with progestin (which is a synthetic version of progesterone).

Methods of Hormone Therapy

There are two methods of administering hormone therapy. They are:

1. Systemic Hormone Therapy

With systemic hormone therapy, the hormones are released into your bloodstream, where they travel to areas of your body where you need it the most. Systemic HT can be administered through:

- Vaginal rings
- Topical formulas that are absorbed through the skin, like gels, creams, sprays, and patches
- Pills
- Low-Dose Vaginal Products

As the name suggests, low-dose vaginal products administer smaller amounts of hormones to the specific area where you are experiencing menopausal symptoms. They usually target menopausal symptoms that affect the urinary tract or the vagina by boosting moisture and thickening up vaginal tissues.

Benefits of Hormone Therapy

- It relieves your menopausal symptoms, including night sweats, hot flashes, vaginal dryness, and even dry and itchy skin
- It reduces health problems associated with a lack of calcium, including osteoporosis and tooth loss. It also reduces your risk of breaking a bone
- Better sense of well-being
- Improved mood
- Reduced risk of developing diabetes
- Reduced risk of colon cancer
- Improved joints and less pain in the joints
- Lower death rate if taken during your 50s
- Reduced risk of dementia and Alzheimer's disease if you begin the therapy during midlife.

Risks of Hormone Therapy

- Increased risk of blood clots
- Increased risk of strokes
- Increased risk of dementia if you begin the therapy after midlife
- Increased risk of developing gallbladder and gallstone problems

- Increased risk of endometrial cancer if you still have your uterus and if you are not taking progestin along with your estrogen
- Increased risk of developing breast cancer if you take it over a long period of time

Your doctor will not recommend HT if you:

- Have had blood clots in the past (or have a family medical history of blood clots)
- Are pregnant or may be pregnant
- Have liver disease
- Have abnormal vaginal bleeding
- Have breast cancer
- Have endometrial cancer
- Have a history of strokes or heart attacks or have a family medical history of vascular disease

Non-Hormonal Therapies

There are non-hormonal, holistic, and medicinal therapies that you can use if HT is not for you.

1. Changing your diet

If you've ever been pregnant or found yourself recovering from an illness, you'll know that it is essential to change your diet to meet your changing dietary needs.

Just think about the last time you had a cold. You probably drank more orange juice and ginger tea. Both contain nutrients that boost the immune system (vitamin C and selenium), giving your body plenty of ammunition to fight off its attackers. The same principle applies to menopause. You can cultivate your diet so that it helps alleviate symptoms of menopause, for example, eating foods with more phytoestrogen, such as ground flax seeds, garlic, berries, wheat bran, and peaches.

Phytoestrogens are plant estrogens that are so similar to human estrogen that they actually work the same when we ingest them. The more phytoestrogen-rich foods you eat, the more estrogen you have circulating around your bloodstream. Once again, I have to say, take that nature!

You will want to eat foods rich in calcium, vitamin D, and magnesium. These nutrients will reduce your chance of developing osteoporosis or even breaking your bones.

If you have a sweet tooth, your doctor will advise you to seriously rein it in once menopause hits. Abdominal fat is associated with diabetes and heart disease, and your chances of gaining abdominal fat and general weight gain increase with menopause.

2. Exercising

Exercising releases feel-good hormones known as endorphins. Endorphins help boost your mood and improve your feelings of well-being. They also reduce your stress and any depression-like feelings you may be experiencing.

Additionally, exercising releases human growth hormone (HGH). HGH maintains blood sugar levels and causes your bones and muscles to grow, also aiding in preventing osteoporosis in mid-age. Regular exercise reduces belly fat and general weight gain caused by menopause.

Don't forget to also add resistance training to your regular workout routine. Resistance training produces testosterone, which increases your muscle mass, improves your bone health, and improves both libido and mood.

3. Avoiding triggers

Eventually, you will notice things that trigger your menopausal symptoms. For example, many women often have particular things that trigger their hot flashes, like heat, smoking, caffeine, spicy food, tight clothing, stress, and so on. Once you can recognize your triggers, avoiding them will bring much relief to your symptoms. If your trigger is tight clothing, you may have to give up thongs for those comfortable briefs, unfortunately! However, with the exercise plan in Chapter Six, you can build a butt so perky it won't even matter!

4. Prescription medications

The FDA has a handy list of menopause medications, including their side effects. You will need to speak to your doctor if you want to try menopause medication. They can prescribe you the best medication that fits your individual medical and menopausal needs.

5. Joining support groups

I'll be honest with you; menopause can be traumatic for some women.

Compounding the issue is that women experience menopause very differently. Some women barely even recognize their symptoms and breeze through it, while some women have to deal with severe symptoms for years. Likewise, in our youth-obsessed culture, it is not psychologically easy to deal with your body changing, signifying your entrance into middle age. Sure, women like Helen Mirren and Michele Obama are now celebrated in our society, but they are still far and few in between. We have a new, progressive tradition battling old stereotypes of older women being useless, unattractive, and cranky.

Sometimes, talking with people who have experienced the same thing you have gives you the courage to carry on. It lets you know you are not alone. Knowing you are not alone in your experiences is such a simple act of connection, yet it is so powerful! It brings you enormous comfort and support and the will to keep going and keep fighting. Ask your healthcare practitioner or local library if they know of any support groups in your area. Luckily, with technology today, you can search for and join online support groups too.

Now that you understand what's going on inside you, you probably feel a weird sense of comfort. This is natural. Accept it and allow it to bring you much-needed healing. Sometimes, knowing the *why* is incredibly important for bringing us relief and comfort. Think back to a hundred years ago, when women had very little medication or medical support for their menopausal symptoms. Then, there was the issue of society's sexism mixed with scientific ignorance. You couldn't even be vocal about your changing body because it was considered impolite and something only a woman of ill morals would do. And, still, women persevered, fought back and won! Today, we can write books about menopause and no one will bat an eye! We can even say the word "menopause" without men fainting around us for daring to bring up a women's health issue! We've come a long way!

Women today are very lucky to have advances in science bring us treatment options that leave us feeling good and looking great! Hurray for female victory! Still, a better option altogether would be not having to go through the pain of menopause.

In the next chapter, we will focus on some of the really challenging symptoms of menopause, namely, night sweats, hot flashes, and insomnia and how to kick their ass, in the name of female victory!

3

ARE THE HOT FLASHES AND INSOMNIA HERE?

You're tossing, and turning, grumpy, irritated, simply trying to sleep. The room is cool, but you feel like a rotisserie chicken turning in the oven. You turn on the AC to full power, however, you've sweat through your bedsheet, and now the damp saturates through to your pajamas. You have an early meeting tomorrow and can't afford to be groggy. Perhaps if you just stay still, sleep will come? Three hours later, you are still awake, and you are still sweating although, thankfully, the hot flashes have gone – for now. If I've not said it before, let me say it now, Welcome to menopause!

In this chapter, we will discuss three particularly pesky menopause symptoms, namely insomnia, hot flashes, and night sweats. I will share with you some not-so-very-secret secrets on how to manage, alleviate and even prevent them, so you can continue to enjoy a good night's rest and a sunshine-filled day, menopause be damned!

HOT FLASHES AND NIGHT SWEATS UNVEILED

Approximately 75%-80% of women suffer from hot flashes. While hot flashes usually begin in peri-menopause, some women actually begin to experience it postmenopause. This is quite common, with many women experiencing a host of menopausal symptoms beginning in postmenopause. Nevertheless, regardless of how severe their hot flashes get, only about 20-30% of women seek medical attention for their symptoms.

Despite our reproductive health being so central to our lives and our overall health, women hardly talk about the negative symptoms of our reproductive system. The ones that do are routinely dismissed, shushed, or told they are overexaggerating. The idea is that women have gone through menopause for centuries, so why would you think you are important enough to want more for yourself? Suck it up, like other women have, and get on with it!

As we have discussed so far in this book, women today are increasingly advocating for change. In the meantime, for those women who are going through menopause in modern society, things like support groups and reading books like this one, help immensely. In the next chapter, we will discuss in more depth how to stay mentally strong through the ups and downs of menopause. For now, let's stick to understanding the science of hot flashes, night sweats and insomnia. Once we understand how these symptoms work scientifically, we can then get a better understanding of how they affect our emotional health and how we can prevent them from doing so in the future.

Hot Flashes

Hot flashes are the most common symptom of menopause. Unfortunately, they also suck the most. Ironically, scientists don't actually know what exactly causes them. They just theorize it has something to do with low estrogen levels or perhaps menopausal changes in the part of the brain that is responsible for controlling bodily temperature.

Imagine sitting under the nice breezy shade of a tree. You feel good. Your skin is breathing, and your body's temperature is at a cool level. Then, suddenly, out of nowhere, the sun travels millions of miles across the universe to sit right next to you! Naturally, you feel an intense, uncomfortable, painful heat. You begin sweating profusely and your skin is red and flushed. Afterward, you feel a strange sense of chill that's just as horrible as the heat. That horrific anecdote defines hot flashes in a nutshell. If you are lucky, your hot flashes may not feel as intense and severe. If you're *really* lucky, you'll be one of those women who experiences very mild symptoms, or very infrequent and short flashes. What we can say, scientifically, however, is that all hot flashes suck! #allhotflashessuck

British actor, Julie Walters, said this about hot flashes: "Oh, God! It was like a chimney and came from the base of my spine. I was doing this TV show called *Murder*, and every take there'd be, 'Stop! She's having a flush!'. At the National, I'd come offstage for a quick change and have to shout, 'Garth, the *tray*!' And this guy would come with this big tin tray and fan me... I was in a wig and padding, and they had to put this big tube of air conditioning in my face!"

On average, hot flashes last between 1-2 minutes, but they can last for up to 10 minutes for some women. Quick tip, if you're one of the really lucky women I've talked about this far in this section, keep it to yourself when dishing about menopause with your girlfriends. It's just not worth it to ruin your friendships over hot flashes! So, when your girlfriend talks about how horrible her symptoms are, just say, "Girl, me too!" and save your friendship in the process!

Hot flashes are such a weird experience and feel differently for different women that it's hard to really describe how it feels, so technically, you won't be lying *per se* to your girlfriend. These tips, and many more, will all be available in my next book, *How to Use Sociopathy to Keep Your Friends*.

Okay, so maybe I'm not really writing that book, but with all jokes aside you will want to familiarize yourself with these common signs of hot flashes:

- Suddenly feeling warmth or even hotness spreading through your face, neck, and chest
- Flushed, red blotchy skin
- Feeling anxious
- Perspiring excessively, especially on your upper body
- Rapid heartbeat
- A chilled feeling as your hot flash ends
- Tingling in your fingers

Night Sweats

Night sweats are just as the name describes. They occur at night, causing you to sweat excessively while asleep. As you can imagine, they severely impact your quality of sleep. Being drenched in sweat is not exactly the best condition for a good night's rest. In fact, some women experience night sweats so profusely that it soaks through their bedding and they have to change it.

Night sweats are not a serious health condition. However, consistently losing sleep can lead to serious health conditions, such as depression, anxiety, and even heart problems.

Night sweats are accompanied by symptoms of hot flashes and typically begin during perimenopause, although they sometimes begin during menopause.

Triggers of Hot Flashes and Night Sweats

Like all menopausal symptoms, hot flashes and night sweat triggers are different for each individual. What triggers you might not trigger your friend and what triggers your friend might not trigger you. If you find these triggers exacerbate or bring on hot flashes and night sweats, then it is best to reduce or cut them out completely:

- Caffeine
- Alcohol
- Hot temperatures/Heat
- Smoking
- Hot/Spicy foods

- Tight clothing/Excess bedding

Try to dress in loose, layered clothing. If you begin to feel a hot flash or a night sweat episode coming on, you can take off layers. Likewise, keep your bed as sparse as possible, to improve airflow and circulation and keep you cool.

- **Stress/Anxiety**

Avoid things that cause you stress and anxiety, including husbands, children, grandchildren, and bosses. If this is not possible and you are not able to find a good hitman or hideout, try to reduce your stress and anxiety levels by eating healthy, exercising often, stretching, getting enough sleep, relaxing, taking time to have fun, spending time with friends and by yourself and practicing your favorite hobbies.

Practicing regular deep breathing exercises will also help you shoo away stress and anxiety. They are also cheaper than hiring a hitman. Not that I know from personal experience or anything like that.

- **Low-High intensity activities**

Sometimes, just going about doing your daily activities can be enough to trigger a hot flash. It's all well and good to say avoid high-intensity activities, but when hot flashes are triggered by unpacking your groceries or preparing a healthy salad for lunch, then we have a problem. Perhaps a better thing to say would be, "Avoid every activity whatsoever on Earth and just breathe." There we go! Problem solved!

- **Drug use**

Drugs can trigger hot flashes. If you are struggling with drug addiction, speak to your doctor to find sources for help.

- **Being overweight/obese**

Being overweight/obese can increase the frequency and intensity of menopause symptoms. Speak with a healthcare professional for professional long-term advice on losing weight healthily. And don't forget to check out my other books on weight loss!

- **Mindfulness meditation**

Meditation, including mindfulness meditation, is a good form of escape, allowing you to escape daily stressors and to tap back into a state of peace and calm.

Managing Hot Flashes

Like all other symptoms of perimenopause and menopause, you can manage hot flashes and night sweats using the following holistic and medical treatment options below. Still, ensure to consult with your doctor before starting any new treatments.

• **Non-hormonal medications**

There are some non-hormonal medications that women experiencing hot flashes and night sweats have had luck with. These include red clover isoflavone extract, vitamin D, evening primrose oil, and soy isoflavone extract.

Additionally, the FDA U.S. Food and Drug Administration has approved the use of the antidepressant paroxetine, although there are other antidepressants that your doctor may be able to prescribe you. Paroxetine is an antidepressant that can be used to treat hot flashes.

It is strongly recommended that you seek a doctor's approval before beginning any of the mentioned medications.

• **Hormones**

Your doctor will be able to assess if you are right for the use of hormone therapy as a treatment for reducing the frequency and intensity of your hot flashes. Your medical history and family's medical history will be assessed to determine if you will benefit from HT. Newer hormone therapy formulations come with less health risks and more health benefits for improving your hot flashes and night sweat symptoms, so hooray for goodness!

Like non-hormonal medication, hormone therapy comes with health risks too, so speak with your doctor about any concerns you may have before you begin HT.

- **Lifestyle changes**

The following lifestyle changes will help you manage your hot flashes:

- Limiting alcohol intake
- Maintaining a lower room temperature than usual
- Maintaining a healthy weight
- Dressing in layers that can be removed at the start of a hot flash
- Exploring mind-body practices, such as yoga, meditation, mindfulness, and tai-chi, to help you stay in tune with your body, so you can recognize the beginning of a hot flash early on and treat it before it overwhelms you
- Exercising

- Sipping ice water at the start of a hot flash
- Keeping a cold pack on your bedside table to use at the beginning of a hot flash
- Using compact pillows that won't trap heat while you sleep
- Avoiding the use of memory foam, since they trap heat
- Using a cooling mattress topper and cooling bed sheets

• Keeping fit

Hot flashes and night sweat symptoms can be alleviated through exercise, particularly exercise that increases your body temperature. Research has shown that consistent exercise over a minimum of 16 weeks reduces the quantity and intensity of hot flashes.

Hot Flash Emergency Kit

You can put together a "hot flash emergency kit" to take with you when you are not at home. You can put this kit in your handbag (if you are one of those women who carries one of those unbelievably large bags for no reason at all). You can also put a kit in your car, one in your office and anywhere else you frequently spend time. Seriously though, what is up with those extra-extra-large bags? I feel like there is some hidden secret network of women with large bags, and I am not privy to their super-important, large-bag secret!

Your hot flash emergency kit should contain: a change of clothes, a change of underwear, a rechargeable hand fan or manual hand fan, water, wipes, tampons and pads, deodorant, toothbrush, spritzer bottle, and maybe even some makeup in case sweating from your hot flash ruins your makeup.

INSOMNIA: THE NO-SLEEP SAGA

Insomnia is characterized by having severe difficulty falling asleep and staying asleep, occurring more than three nights each week. Insomniacs usually suffer from restless sleep, low-quality sleep, and waking up way too early in the morning without being able to fall back asleep. Consequently, insomniacs are usually fatigued, cranky, and sleepy all day. According to Harvard Health, "Sleep disturbances such as insomnia are extremely common, especially in women after menopause. According to data from the National Institutes of Health, sleep disturbance varies from 16% to 42% before menopause, from 39% to 47% during perimenopause, and from 35% to 60% after menopause."

Our hormones control our sleep. Since we experience hormonal imbalance during menopause, this change in hormonal levels can result in insomnia. Likewise, constantly waking up because of other menopause symptoms, such as night sweats and frequent urination, can eventually lead to insomnia. Indeed, insomnia, in some cases, can be psychological. Since menopause is such a pivotal time in a woman's life, it is possible to carry a lot of unresolved emotions about your experience that then unwittingly keep you awake.

Still, insomnia is not just caused by perimenopause and menopause. Some of it is due to aging. As we grow older, we produce less melatonin. Melatonin is a small molecule in our body responsible for making us sleepy at night. It regulates our sleep rhythm and is found in different parts of the body, including the placenta, the gut, and the ovaries.

Another cause of insomnia related to aging is sleep-disordered breathing, namely sleep apnea and snoring. These can wake you up periodically, in particular, if you suffer from obstructive sleep apnea, a sleep disorder that is characterized by temporary pauses in your breathing. These pauses cause you to jolt back to breathing, leading to snoring, gasping for air, choking, and waking up numerous times throughout the night. Unfortunately, research shows that once you begin perimenopause, your risk of developing sleep apnea increases by four percent every year. Sleep apnea is thought to be caused by lower progesterone levels.

If you suffer from other conditions that prevent sleep, such as restless leg syndrome and periodic limb movements disorder, then you may very well develop insomnia, particularly when these conditions are combined with other menopausal symptoms that disrupt sleep.

Insomnia is a serious condition that must not be taken lightly. Our bodies need sleep like fish need water and middle-aged men need fedoras and flat caps! Seriously, what is up with middle-aged men and their love of middle-aged guy hats? I guess fedoras and flat caps are to middle-aged men like extra large bags are to grown women.

Without sleep, our physical, mental, and emotional health rapidly deteriorate. As such, it is not uncommon for people suffering from insomnia to develop depression, anxiety, or even suicide ideation. Insomnia also impairs focus and memory and increases inflammation in the body, all symptoms which just suck the fun out of life.

Remedies for Insomnia

Luckily, there are treatments for insomnia. Usually, by combining two or more treatments, you can beat this condition! All you and your doctor need are a period of trial and error until you find which ones work best for you.

Remedies for insomnia include:

• Yoga and exercise

Yoga is a particularly great remedy for insomnia. It relies on deep breathing exercises and deep stretches and twists to release your joints and muscles, promoting deep relaxation throughout your body and creating perfect conditions for deep sleep. Yoga exercises can also improve the strength of your pelvic floor, allowing you to sleep through the night without needing to get up to use the toilet. Strong pelvic floor exercises also improve sex, so get to doing your Kegels and yoga!

Yoga encourages you to let go of your thoughts and worries and to simply breathe deeply and be present in the moment. It promotes mental calm and clarity, creating the right conditions for falling asleep. Avoid yoga that gets your heart pumping just before bed. In particular, avoid hot yoga and vinyasa flow styles, as these are high-energy, high-intensity yoga styles that energize you too much before bed. You want to be sleepy and feeling good, not wide awake and feeling like you can take on a bear in a fight!

As well as yoga, you should do regular medium-high intensity exercises for thirty minutes three times a day. I dare you to spend one afternoon this week going on a brisk walk, lifting weights, or going on a high-incline walk on your treadmill. Then, when you get home at night, try to stay awake for the next three hours. You'll find it almost impossible. Why? Because these are medium-high-intensity exercises that tire you out.

Exercise causes your muscles to tear. To repair themselves and become stronger and bigger, your muscles need sleep. Naturally, since you spend all your energy exercising, your brain releases hormones and chemicals, like melatonin to make you fall asleep so that your body can repair itself. In a lot of ways, exercise is like the perfect drug. It makes you feel good, it can be cheap and still work, it increases your confidence, it makes life seem brighter and better, and it releases endorphins, which literally gives you the sensation of being high, by promoting a feeling of euphoria and by having a sedative effect on you! It's a shame exercise requires discipline, otherwise it would be a really popular drug.

Similarly, exercise improves your quality of life in so many ways, one or more of these are bound to improve your sleep too. For instance, the more you exercise, the more you lose weight. The more you lose weight, the more you decrease your risk of developing sleep apnea, thereby improving your sleep.

• Supplements

While you can get many of your nutrients from a healthy, balanced diet, scientists say that our food today contains fewer nutrients than food of the past. Hence, you may need supplements to ensure you are getting enough of the right nutrients. If you exercise a lot, particularly high-intensity exercises, your daily required amount of nutrients also increases, meaning that you may not be able to get all your nutrients from food alone.

If you feel you would benefit from taking supplements, speak with your doctor, who will be able to determine what nutrients you may be deficient in, as well as how much of those nutrients you need to take in supplement form.

Speak with your doctor about the possibility of using the supplements below, which are known for promoting good sleep:

- Multivitamins
- Magnolia bark

- Magnesium

• Hormone therapy

As with hot flashes and night sweats, hormone therapy can correct some of the hormonal imbalances in your body leading to insomnia.

• Diet

Your main source of nutrients comes from your diet. In turn, your diet determines, in some part, the hormones your body produces and how much of those hormones it produces. For example, premenopausal women who ingest a lot of sugar in their diet produce an overabundance of estrogen. This estrogen overabundance then affects many of their bodily functions, leading to health conditions.

Your diet is even more important in perimenopause and menopause because it can be a way to balance out some of your hormonal imbalances. Or, at the very least, to relieve symptoms of menopause. For instance, a low-GI diet has been shown to reduce the risk of developing insomnia, particularly for menopausal and perimenopausal women. Chapter Eight will take you on a magical journey, giving you nutrition and health tips for the modern menopausal woman. It ends with a

28-day weight loss meal plan, so you can feel good, look good, and give menopause the finger!

• Aromatherapy

Have you ever walked by a lavender garden in summer? The flowers' wonderful fragrance is perfumed around the air, making you feel as though you've just walked through a fairytale. You continue walking by, a smile on your face, only to realize a few seconds later that you feel rejuvenated! Another five seconds later, you let out a big sigh that seems to drain all the stress and anxiety from the deepest regions of your soul! That power that the flowers possess is the power of aromatherapy.

I used to have a menopausal client who was having serious difficulty with her sleeping. She was quite unfortunate because she had tried almost everything with no success. She had suffered from insomnia for decades before menopause even began, so it was clear that menopause was making a bad situation worse. One day, as she shared with me her difficulties with insomnia, I stopped and remembered a practice I had learned.

The routine involved lighting relaxing incense sticks or burning fragrance candles, turning off the lights, setting the temperature in the room to a very comfortable (warm/cold) degree, listening to some relaxing yoga songs, and then doing some deep yoga stretches. This routine is meant to relax the mind and set you off into a relaxing sleep. My client was skeptical, but she agreed to try it. She was so grateful when it worked for her!

Aromatherapy is a wonderful way of tapping into your mental state and elevating your mood. Since sleep problems can be rooted in our mental states and our moods, aromatherapy can help you tap into the deeper recesses of your subconscious and unconscious. Breathing calms anxiety and unresolved feelings, thus alleviating your sleep problems and restoring emotional balance.

One research study published in the *Journal of Menopausal Medicine* confirms that aromatherapy may be beneficial in improving the psychological symptoms among menopausal women. Some of the best scents for sleep are:

- Chamomile
- Lavender
- Sandalwood
- Cedarwood
- Marjoram
- Bergamot

You will also want to consider avoiding caffeine, nicotine, and alcohol. Caffeine is notorious for keeping us awake, so even little traces of caffeine in our system can make insomnia symptoms worse. You may need to give up coffee for something with less caffeine in it, like green tea. Alcohol and nicotine also make it difficult for you to sleep, so quit, girl! Now, that's easier said than done, so if you find it difficult to quit, speak with a healthcare professional to find out the options available to you to help you on this journey.

The best way to discover and manage your triggers is to keep a "trigger journal." Wherever you deal with hot flashes, night sweats, and insomnia, write down all the things you ate, wore, and did hours and even days before the episode. This will help you to track potential triggers and identify patterns and conditions that accompany or cause your symptoms. The more you can find specific triggers, the better you can avoid them and reduce the frequency and intensity of your symptoms, allowing you to feel great for longer!

There are two things you can't buy in this life: good health and peace. Perimenopause and menopause can be stealers of your good health and peace. They act like haters, annoyed and jealous because you enjoy good sleep every night, wake up without dark circles, and don't suffer from any hot flashes or night sweats. So they plan your downfall like two evil divas trying to take down the Queen Bee.

Nevertheless, you can't ever really take down the Queen. She may be temporarily defeated but she always returns to claim her crown! You can still take back your health and peace from menopause using your one weapon in your arsenal: your trigger journal. Then, as soon as you have identified your triggers, it's simply a matter of finding treatments that work to defeat each symptom.

You may be lucky and find that the first few treatments you try are successful. Conversely, you may need to try a few treatments and a few combinations of treatments before you find one that works for you. Don't give up hope. Be resilient in your pursuit of peace and good health. Remember that some women experience menopausal symptoms even into their postmenopausal years, so the earlier you can find treatments that work, the quicker you can get back to being you again and the quicker you can get back to feeling and looking great.

You're a queen, and queens always look great! It's a great tactic for intimidating your enemies, i.e., peri-menopause and menopause, so put your Ruby Woo lipstick on, brush your hair, and find those triggers!

In the next chapter, we will concentrate on how menopause affects women's mental health. To defeat a queen, you must attack not just her armies but also her spirit. Fierce warriors will follow a great leader to the ends of the Earth. But if you break the Queen's spirit, the warriors have no one to motivate them to victory. In the next chapter, I will teach you how to defend your spirit from your menopausal enemies and protect your mental health and emotional peace from this thief!

Sharpen your sword and join me in the next chapter as we prepare for battle!

4

STAYING MENTALLY STRONG
DURING MENOPAUSE

Shirleen, my friend, was the life of the party. Or, in this case, the life of the gym. She marched in one drab, rainy afternoon, seeking a personal trainer. We all fell in love with her wit, confidence, and her love of life. She drew us in so completely that she just became good friends with all of us. She was always smiling, always happy, and always determined to lift people's spirits.

We were all very happy when she was around because she just seemed to spread joy with her presence. It seemed as though everyone around her became happier when she was around - even the people who didn't know her!

A few years after Shirleen became a regular at the gym (and a pretty popular one at that), she casually informed me that she had begun perimenopause. We spent some time changing her diet and exercise plan to meet her changing hormonal needs, and that was that. Nonetheless, a few months later, I noticed that Shirleen had changed. It seemed as though she had just become a different person. Yes, her body had changed as a result of her hormonal imbalance. However, what was most noticeable was the change in her mood. She was exhibiting depression-like symptoms. She rarely smiled or laughed and seemed to want to keep to herself. She had very little energy to work out and, as a result, was gaining weight. Further causing her weight gain was that she seemed unable to follow my instructions or the things I was saying, as though she was trapped in a mental fog.

She then shared with me that she had been battling severe depression and anxiety that came about once she began perimenopause. Her symptoms got so bad she began having thoughts filled with intense despair and hopelessness. Indeed, things have gotten so bad that she quit her job and had to take some time to find a new job. This was when she realized that she had to get medical help.

She eventually went to see her doctor, and they found an antidepressant prescription that works for her. She beamed as she shared with me that she was finally feeling better.

Although I knew that perimenopause and menopause can sometimes trigger depression-like feelings, I will admit that I was still quite naive at how badly some women experience depression and mood disorders, such as anxiety, during this period of their lives. It took Shirlene's experience to really snap me out of this naivete and to really pay attention to the mental health of my perimenopausal and menopausal clients. As a result, I began to plan their exercise and diet plans around improving their mental health symptoms to help them stay mentally strong through menopause.

Shirleen's experience also taught me that menopause can have a severely dark side that most people don't know about, understand, or want to talk about. She had withdrawn into herself because she felt no one would understand or care. Of course, this was partly true since women's menopausal experiences are still routinely ignored by society. Nonetheless, it was also partly untrue. Depression has a way of making you withdraw from those who care about you the most, and Shirleen had many people who cared about her and wanted to help her through her depression. Unfortunately, that very depression caused her to hide away from those who wanted to help her the most. Luckily, Shirleen did eventually reach out to her doctor and to her family. Slowly, she was able to reintegrate into society. Her story is a great reminder to me that women can pull through the darkest days of menopause. In this chapter, we will explore some of the ways to stay mentally strong during the really dark parts of menopause.

There is no need to sugarcoat the fact that menopause can bring really rainy days. Sugarcoating it is only setting you up for failure if those dark days do indeed come. Instead, let us discuss menopausal mental health with an open mind and a willingness to talk about this uncomfortable topic, knowing that it is for our own benefit as women. Like *Sex and the City* actor Kim Catrall said, menopause is not shameful but is, rather, a natural part of life. "It's as natural as having a child—it really is; it's part of life. Physically, it's part of how we're made; hormonally, it's how we're constructed; chemically, it's how we work. Like anything in nature: The seed is planted, it grows, it comes to fruition, and after a period of time it starts to change and age, and it's scary. You wonder, Will I be attractive, desirable, feminine? What is the next chapter of life? I think it's one of the reasons why it's so taboo is because we don't talk about it—it's too frightening even to talk to a doctor about it. I want to reach out to women to encourage them to educate themselves about this time in their lives."

DOES MENOPAUSE AFFECT MENTAL HEALTH?

According to the website letstalkmenopause.org, "38% of women in late perimenopause report symptoms of depression such as irritability, mood swings & fatigue. The stats are even more shocking when you discover that, women who have never experienced depression are two to four times more likely to experience a depressive episode during the menopausal transition".

Depression

Scientifically speaking, puberty, pregnancy, and menopause are very vulnerable periods of a woman's life because of all the hormonal changes you are going through, affecting your mood, mental health, and emotional health. Indeed, what science does know is that the level of the brain chemical, serotonin, in our body plummets to reflect estrogen's plummeting rate in our bodies. You also know about progesterone from Chapter Two. Well, as it turns out, progesterone works with estrogen to manage neurotransmitters, dopamine and serotonin, two neurotransmitters (that act as hormones) that regulate our mood.

With less estrogen and progesterone, serotonin and dopamine levels in your body also fall. Ultimately, this means they can't do their jobs as well as they used to, and your risk of developing depression and other mood disorders increases. Since these two neurotransmitters also regulate your mood, low levels of serotonin and dopamine result in mood swings. You also feel less able to cope with daily stressors that wouldn't have bothered you pre-menopause, hence you begin to experience irritability, anxiety, and increased stress.

Serotonin is also responsible for improving your feelings of well-being and happiness. That's why being out in the sunshine increases your feelings of happiness. Scientists believe that the human skin may be capable of generating serotonin when you are out in the sunshine. This is also why some people develop seasonal affective disorder (SAD) during the winter months when there is barely any sunshine. Known as the "feel-good" chemical, serotonin keeps you emotionally stable and mentally focused. When it comes to sleep, serotonin works together with dopamine to give you good quality, deep sleep. (It's also why you fall asleep after Thanksgiving dinner. Turkey contains large quantities of tryptophan, which your body uses to make serotonin.) Serotonin and dopamine also work together to increase your libido, which is why people battling depression often see a decrease in their libido. It all pretty much boils down to how important serotonin is for preventing mood disorders in our bodies and how hormonal changes in our bodies during menopause make it difficult for serotonin to do its job.

If you experienced a period of major depression in the past, you are at a higher risk of developing it during perimenopause and menopause. Additionally, other symptoms of menopause, such as insomnia, hot flashes, night sweats, and urinary incontinence disrupt your sleep. Difficulty sleeping, regular sleep disturbances, and poor sleep quality all increase your chances of developing depression by up to ten times.

Just when you think the depressing part is over (no pun intended), there's more. In order to be an even bigger life disrupter and winner of the award for "Most Likely to Overturn Your Life Negatively," perimenopause and menopause also invite themselves into your life during a very turbulent period: middle age. In middle age, our lives change at a rapid pace. Women deal with kids leaving home, divorcing husbands or breaking up with partners, finding new partners, looking after aging parents, becoming grandparents, pressures from their careers, and other health problems not associated with perimenopause and menopause. So, not only are you having to deal with coming home every night to a now-empty nest, you also have to find money in an already too-tight budget to take care of your aging father, while battling ageism in the workplace and problems in your marriage that you do not know how to fix. With less serotonin and dopamine, climbing Mount Everest naked, without your glasses, seems like a better time than dealing with these stressors. You no longer have the hormonal and chemical balance to help you deal with it all, leaving you vulnerable to becoming depressed or anxious.

Speak with your doctor if you have any of these symptoms of depression:

- Insomnia or oversleeping
- Thoughts of suicide
- Overwhelming fatigue that you can't shake
- Lack of motivation
- Not eating much or overeating
- Feeling hopelessness and sadness persistently
- Consistent irritability
- Having no interest in things that you used to enjoy
- Difficulty absorbing information
- Difficulty making decisions

If you notice you are experiencing depression symptoms that are getting in the way of your day-to-day life at home and at work and have lasted for more than two weeks, seek help immediately! This could be from a doctor, family member, friend, or anyone you trust. You don't have to reach out to your doctor first. What's more important is that you simply reach out to someone you trust. They may then be able to support you with booking an appointment with your doctor and accompanying you to that appointment.

Stress and Anxiety

Menopause isn't exactly a walk on the beach. Going through night sweats that have kept you up all night, then blanking out during an important business meeting the next day, only to go home extremely tired and unable to sleep due to insomnia. On top of that, most women are going through big life changes at this point in their life, whether it be divorce, dating, welcoming a grandchild, kids leaving home, semi-retiring, etc. This simply equates to more deadlines, more calls and messages to respond to, more expectations, more people relying on you, and less time for yourself or your health.

Stress only breeds anxiety, and anxiety only breeds stress. The two feed off of each other, growing bigger and stronger, until they overwhelm you. You may even get to a point where you begin to worry about when the next menopause symptom will appear and whether it will uproot or change your life!

The best way to defeat stress is through your mindset. When the expectations, deadlines, responsibilities, and persevering through your symptoms finally get to you, remind yourself that stress is a normal part of life. You will always be stressed, so why let it win every single time? Since you will always have something to stress about, isn't it better to just let the weight roll off you instead of pressing you down? You can choose to be deliberate in choosing laughter and positivity when the negativity of stress wants to overwhelm you. Physically, you can choose to eat healthy since this reinforces your brain and nervous system against many of the effects of stress and anxiety on the body. Speak with your doctor about using adaptogens like ashwagandha and maca root. (Adaptogens are plants and mushrooms that fortify your body against the effects of stress, anxiety, and fatigue and promote a general sense of well-being.) You can also use herbs and teas to promote a sense of calm. For example, there is nothing I crave more after a hard grueling day than a nice hot chamomile tea, to cover me with that wonderful overall sense of well-being that I felt as a child on Christmas Eve - back when I still believed in magic and Santa Claus.

For good measure, exercise. I used to have a neighbor who battled depression for years. Hoping to be prescribed medication, her doctor advised her to go on regular long walks. At first it seemed she was sceptical but, a year later, she shared with me how she was no longer depressed.

According to the American Psychological Association, "many experts believe routine exercise is as powerful in treating anxiety and mood disorders as antidepressants. Preliminary evidence suggests that physically active people have lower rates of anxiety and depression than sedentary people. Psychologists also recommend exercise to their patients because it leads to a sense of accomplishment. Getting dressed and driving to the gym first thing in the morning may not be so fun in the moment, but prioritizing self-care practices like exercise can result in a cascade effect of other healthy habits, like eating nutritiously, socializing with others, and getting a good night's sleep — all of which can improve depression symptoms."

You will notice that exercise is mentioned more than a few times in this book. That's because the benefits of exercise are so much that it really is one of the best forms of self-care you can do for your body.

Panic Attacks

In the same article cited above, the American Psychological Association shares that exercising is a good practice for learning how to respond to panic attacks because our bodies have similar responses to panic attacks as they do exercise. Essentially, exercise is a multipurpose menopause-busting tool! If you haven't already, it's time to get shopping to add a few workout gear to your wardrobe! Maybe even buy that hot pink crop top! Why not? You only live once, and menopause isn't going to stop you from looking like eye candy!

Panic attacks are copycats of stress and anxiety. They are more likely to show up in response to the upheaval menopause brings. Like stress, if you are having a panic attack, it helps tremendously if you practice acceptance. Breathe and tell yourself, *"This is just a normal reaction to the upheaval in my life. It's nothing to worry about. It will pass."* Take really deep breaths as you allow the attack to run its course without ascribing any negativity to the experience. Panic attacks are like naughty children throwing a tantrum. Paying them negative attention is still attention. Act as though this is normal and it doesn't bother you, and the panic attack will end much quicker.

You can also try using a mindfulness meditation technique known as "grounding." Grounding involves intensely focusing on an object, person, or any other stimuli around you. For instance, you can look at your partner and the ridiculous mustache he's been growing out "to try a new look." To intensely focus on the mustache, you pay attention to every piece of information you can take in about this ridiculous tache. Focus on the texture, color, length, whether it looks soft or bristle, how it makes you feel, anything it reminds you of, like your Uncle Carl's epically manly mustache - now *that* was a mustache to rival all mustaches! The more you pay attention to the mustache, the more you are not paying any attention to the panic attack. The more you are not paying any attention to the panic attack, the more it does not affect you and fizzles out. It's sort of like encountering a poisonous snake. The more you don't pay attention to the snake … Actually, this might be a bad analogy because the snake will bite you regardless. The point is, to defeat panic attacks, pay attention to something else.

Marital or Relationship Stress

Although your partner's terrible mustache might be objectively terrible, the great news with menopause is you might not even be able to judge accurately because you are battling irritability. It very well could be a fine mustache, but your hormones are all over the place, making you see it as a monstrosity.

Unfortunately, irritability is not the only issue. Depression, fatigue, stress, anxiety, panic attacks, weight gain, and even health conditions resulting from menopause would drive anyone crazy. It gets so bad for some women that their irritability is taken out as rage on unsuspecting loved ones. It's no surprise that menopause tends to put a strain on women's personal relationships. Women in this situation can often feel misunderstood, isolated, and socially excluded. They feel deep guilt and shame for acting this way since they are generally nice, collected, and emotionally well-regulated women.

If you find menopause to be placing a strain on your personal relationships, you can try attending counseling with the other person(s). You can also try to educate your loved ones about the natural effects of menopause and what to expect so they are not surprised by changes in your behavior.

Perceived Cognitive Decline

Menopausal symptoms are like your partner's terrible mustache. It refuses to go away! (You gave it more thought on a day when you weren't feeling irritable and concluded the mustache was objectively terrible.) Just when you pat yourself on the back for dealing with one symptom with the royal class of Lady Diana, another one shows up, ready to ruin your week. This time, it's perceived cognitive decline.

Notice the use of the word "perceived" at the beginning. That's because what you really go through is cognitive impairment. Sudden changes in your hormonal balance, especially in your estrogen levels, also disrupt the way your brain works. As a result, you experience things like walking into a room and forgetting what you came in for, slower thinking, confusion or difficulty concentrating on your supermarket run, and forgetting to buy your partner's facial hair cream, hoping that would make it all fall off (wink wink).

What's important to remember is that cognitive impairment is temporary. Once your body begins to regulate its hormonal state again, you will notice an improvement. And, if you need to, you can always use hormone therapy to improve your cognitive performance.

AM I EXPERIENCING MENTAL HEALTH ISSUES?

Mental health is a very complex subject. Moreover, anyone can experience mental health issues at any time and for any reason, including no reason at all. Of course, menopause increases your risk of experiencing mental health issues since estrogen is pivotal in promoting good mental health.

Nonetheless, it's pretty common for women to be uncertain about whether their symptoms can be classified as a mental health issue. Compounding this is the fact that, let's face it, many women put up with a lot of behaviors that affect our mental health because we feel as though no one would really care if we spoke our truths. Even pre-menopause, we may have felt depressed, sad, anxious, unappreciated, taken-for-granted, bullied, disrespected, and a host of negative emotions that are sometimes birthed from sexism. What menopause then does is exaggerate the negative feelings that we already had anyway, causing confusion as to what is going on with our mental health and what can or cannot be ascribed to menopause.

We have already examined many signs of mental health issues you may experience during menopause. To help you clarify it, here is a simplified list of symptoms you may experience if you are having mental health issues.

- An increase in your drug or alcohol use

Using drugs to cope with mental health issues is very common and is usually a classic sign that you have mental health issues that need to be addressed in a healthy manner.

- Irritability

"Your. Partner's. Mustache. Needs. To. Be. Shaved. Now!"

Irritability, anger, and rage targeted toward those closest to you are classic menopausal symptoms. It can lead to a swift deterioration in your relationships, which, in turn, leads to further mental health issues. Always remember that this irritability is not your fault, but it is your body's way of reacting to hormonal changes. Our bodies, unfortunately, react to our hormones even before our conscious brain can take over. It's the same reason why hungry people are hangry and act as though they want to slap everyone around them. That is, until you throw a donut at their face! They're not bad people, and you're not a bad person! It really is just human hormones making us all act like big bad wolves!

- Increased worry or anxiety

Use grounding and acceptance exercises when worry and anxiety grip you. This will allow the wave of anxiety to pass by much quicker.

- Low motivation or energy

Estrogen energizes us. Without it, we feel depleted. Without estrogen, we are also more likely to become depressed. Low motivation and energy is a typical sign of depression. Dealing with other mental health issues also brings down our motivation for life, leaving us listless and wondering, "What's the point?" If you feel like your motivation and energy levels are low, speak with your doctor to find treatment options to help fix the issue.

- Thoughts of death or suicide

This is common when experiencing depression and should be taken extremely seriously. Reach out to someone immediately if you have thoughts of death or suicide.

- Mood swings

Eat nutrient-rich foods, exercise often, sleep well, practice mindfulness meditation, and treat yourself once in a while. While this won't completely prevent all mood swings, it will reduce the frequency. If you experience frequent mood swings, speak with your doctor about using hormone therapy. Or alternatively, you can ask your doctor about using supplements and adaptogens to promote a general sense of well-being.

An apology and explanation also goes a long way. Apologize to those in the line of fire during your mood swings and ask them to throw a donut at you during your next episode to snap you out of it. Then you can take the rational step to go for a walk, practice some grounding exercises, or do anything else that will help you channel that energy out, so it is not being channeled at others in a way that can be harmful to them.

- Persistent feelings of pessimism, guilt, worthlessness, bitterness, or anger

It's not easy dealing with your emotions when your hormones are imbalanced. Many women feel a deep sense of guilt, shame, and fear because their mood swings and irritability cause them to lash out in ways that could be considered abusive to others. It is always best to explain to people you come in contact with regularly that you are going through menopause and that some irritability and mood swings are to be expected. We tend to allow pregnant women off the hook when they act "crazy" because we all accept their hormones are practicing acrobatics inside them. If you explain to people it's kind of like the mood swings a pregnant woman experiences, they will understand and will cut you some slack. If, on the other hand, you meet a person who refuses to be understanding, well, not everyone you meet will be open-minded. Try throwing a donut at their head to open their mind, but maybe just visualize doing it as a grounding technique because you don't want to get sued for assault by donut.

As well as feelings of guilt and shame, you may also experience rage and anger alongside your irritability. You may also experience feelings of worthlessness, bitterness, and pessimism. These are normal and nothing to worry about. If they persist for months, speak to your doctor about treatment options.

Other symptoms that can point to mental health issues are:

- A noticeable increase or decrease in your appetite and weight
- Feeling overwhelmed
- Crying more than normal
- Not feeling like yourself
- Difficulty concentrating
- Socially isolating yourself from others

Typically, you will notice more than one symptom. It has something to do with our brains, nervous system, and hormones just being this huge supercomputer with so many interconnected parts that make it likely for you to experience a symptom or two that point towards mental health issues even though you might not actually be going through a mental health issue.

For example, since I am a personal trainer, I exercise regularly. This means my metabolism is really fast. It also means that once I deplete my glucose levels, my stomach secretes an insane amount of the hormone ghrelin, and I begin to exhibit mental health issues, like feeling incredibly sad, feeling that the world is just an awful place, feeling overwhelmed, and being incredibly irritable (i.e. hangry). Then I eat my lunch, and the world is all sunshine, lollipops, fairies, and cute puppies! It would be easy for me to mistake my hangriness for a mental health issue, when it was just my brain computer reacting to low blood glucose with symptoms of mental health issues.

Another way to ascertain that you are indeed dealing with symptoms of mental health issues, and not something else, is through the length of time these symptoms last. My symptoms tend to last until I munch on my delicious Falafel Avocado Wrap; then, I no longer feel as though I hate my coworkers! That is clearly not a sign of mental health issues since all it takes is a lunch break to make my two-hour symptoms disappear. When you are dealing with symptoms of mental health issues, they typically last for weeks and months and don't disappear with something as simple as one good meal or a tasty donut.

RISK FACTORS

As with all things mental health, there are certain risk factors that increase your likelihood of developing mental health issues, namely:

- Lack of social and emotional support

Did you know that one factor that decides whether a person will develop PTSD after a traumatic event is whether or not they receive the right social and emotional support after the event? With the right social and emotional support, humans have this amazing ability to be able to survive some really dark days and go on to heal and thrive afterward. Certainly, this isn't the only factor determining if a person will survive or heal from a painful experience, but it is an important determining factor nonetheless.

For example, if you have family members who are able to meet you halfway and throw a donut or slice of bread at your head when irritability strikes, despite how ludicrous that sounds, it shows you that they love you enough to let go of any negative emotions your rage and irritability might cause them and still tap into themselves to respond with the positive emotions you need to pull you out of your negative emotional state. This makes you feel supported and loved, which, in turn, allows for the release of the love hormone, "dopamine."

Dopamine is a powerful "reward" neurotransmitter/hormone that can help us feel good and regulate our mood. To get a sense of how pleasurable dopamine feels, imagine petting your dog or cat while the scent of cinnamon fills your warm home. It's snowing heavily outside, and it looks like a Christmas card from beyond your window. Indoors, the apples are bubbling up from the pie crust baking in the oven, and your favorite songs are playing. You are wrapped up in your partner's arms while sipping on hot cocoa with perhaps a little too much sugar, and your bank app just sent a notification to say you just got paid! Picture how great you would feel in that moment. Well, that feeling is caused by dopamine.

The more emotional and social support we receive, the more our brains produce dopamine. Since dopamine regulates functions in our bodies, such as sleep, mood, focus, attention, and pain processing, it can nullify and alleviate some menopausal symptoms, reducing your likelihood of developing mental health issues. For those symptoms you do experience, dopamine is also able to wipe over the pain they cause with pleasure, making you less likely to develop mental health issues. Conversely, for women who don't experience the dopamine release triggered by good social and emotional support, their likelihood of developing mental health issues increases.

- Experiencing major life changes or challenges during the menopause transition

Stress is kind of like lifting weights. We all have a maximum amount of weight that we can lift without messing up our backs. Some people are naturally stronger and can lift more. Others train, becoming stronger and more resilient so they can lift heavier weights. And some people just don't have the physique to lift weights and are better suited to activities like yoga, ballet, swimming, or eating cake on the couch. Menopause is already very stressful, even for women who only experience mild symptoms. Not only is it physically stressful, it is also mentally and emotionally stressful. You have to deal with the existential question of what life means to you in middle age. Then, many women have to deal with accepting the loss of their youth and the loss of the privilege that comes with having youth in a youth-obsessed society. This is not to mention the emotional stress of feeling as though your symptoms are ruining your relationships.

In short, menopause has you carrying your maximum amount of stress weight. Experiencing a major life change or challenge during this period is the equivalent of someone adding 50 lbs to your weight bar. If you have good social and emotional support, they could rally around to help you carry it (see how I cleverly intertwined all three metaphors together)? If you have been through past stressful events and learned techniques and practices for dealing with them, then those muscles could kick in and give you the strength and power you need to carry the extra weight. Still, if you don't have either of these, then you may very well collapse under this heavier weight, causing you to experience mental health issues.

- Lack of positive health behaviors, such as healthy eating or regular engagement in exercise

Since all parts of the human body are connected, the more you take care of each part with care, the healthier your body as a whole is. When one part stops working as normal - in the case of menopause, this would be the production of estrogen - your body might be able to make up for this change if all other functions and parts of your body are in good working condition. Certain parts of your body are so pivotal you can't function without them. Parts like your heart and brain are integral to your entire body working. However, because your body can continue to power on without working ovaries, an overall healthy body will be better equipped to deal with the blow of menopause and to adjust much quicker than a body that is not overall in good healthy condition.

Let's take a particular example specific to menopause. We know that our adrenal glands continue to produce smaller amounts of estrogen during menopause and postmenopause. If you have an unhealthy diet, packed with white sugars, soda, white flour, processed foods, fried foods, and artificial sweeteners, you could experience adrenal fatigue, whereby your adrenal glands are so stressed, that they stop functioning well. If your adrenal glands are fatigued during menopause, this means they may not be able to function well enough to produce those small amounts of estrogen that could be the difference between whether or not you can carry the weight of menopause, or whether the weight becomes too heavy for you.

- Experiencing consistent lack of sleep

Sleep is like oxygen, food, and water. Humans are dependent on it for survival. When it comes to menopause, research has shown that sleep actually improves many menopausal symptoms that women experience. For instance, there is a clear link between sleep and depression. Depression can worsen sleep problems. Sleep problems, in turn, worsen depression, beginning and continuing a cycle that becomes difficult to escape. Research has also shown that people experiencing stress, such as the stress caused by menopause, may experience a decrease in the amount of time spent in deep sleep, and disruptions during REM sleep [an important stage of sleep]. For perimenopausal and menopausal women, sleep is like healthy eating or exercise. It fortifies your emotional and mental resilience towards distressing, painful, and uncomfortable menopausal symptoms.

- Other health issues emerging during this time, especially thyroid issues, which may lead to further hormonal imbalances

Fortunately, your ovaries stopping production of estrogen does not mean all other factories in your body shut down. Hormones still need to be produced! Food still needs to be digested! Leg muscles still need to move! Your brain still needs to process information, and so on. This is great news in the long-term because it illustrates that there is certainly life postmenopause. Unfortunately, it also means you may develop other health issues during this menopausal stage of life. While some issues may not affect menopause too much, for example needing to remove a tooth, others may, in particular, issues that cause hormonal imbalance.

Maintaining hormonal balance in the body is already a complicated thing, even in women who are not menopausal. This is partly to do with our menstrual cycle and partly to do with the human body just having so many hormones performing so many functions that one little twink in the whole production line could cause a breakdown of the entire system. During menopause, there are so many twinks, the entire factory just gets set on fire! Firefighters are called in to do the best they can to put out the fire so it can be rebuilt. Health issues that cause hormonal imbalance (like thyroid issues) are kind of like if the firefighters arrived with diesel in their fire truck instead of water.

The stress of going through two or more health conditions causing hormonal imbalance is phenomenal because your body is acting like its wires have gone completely haywire, you cannot find homeostasis (balance in your entire body and bodily functions), and your discomfort and pain have doubled and maybe even tripled. Naturally, you can see how this can lead to mental health issues for someone going through this.

ALL HOPE IS NOT LOST – IT'S JUST ON A COFFEE BREAK

All hope is not lost. There are treatment options for menopause-related mental health issues, allowing you to continue to be fabulous, sexy, warm, friendly, and any other positive adjective that can be used to describe the wonderfulness of you. If you find yourself despairing over your mental health thanks to menopause, try one (or a combination) of these methods to help relieve your symptoms, so the world can slowly become sunshine, lollipops, fairies, and cute puppies once more!

- Cognitive Behavioral Therapy

According to the British Menopause Society cognitive behavioral therapy can help with a host of menopausal symptoms, from depression, to anxiety, to stress, to hot flushes, night sweats, and sleep problems. Cognitive behavioral therapy is a form of therapy that aids you in developing practical techniques for coping with and managing your emotional and mental reactions to external stimuli and events. With CBT, you learn that you can't necessarily change the external world, but if you learn healthy ways to cope with external stimuli that provoke a negative emotional response, you improve your mental health as a result.

Since the way we think about our symptoms affects how we feel about menopause (which then affects how we react to our mental health), CBT trains you to think about your symptoms in positive and neutral ways, so that your mental health is not being affected. To learn how to use CBT to treat your mental health symptoms of menopause, you will first need to find a therapist. Your therapist will teach you how to use CBT to develop a calmer and more accepting attitude towards your menopausal symptoms, including the mental health symptoms. The general objective of CBT is to teach you that negative reactions to your menopausal symptoms are not facts. Stress, anxiety, negative thinking, and so on, are just one interpretation of your menopausal symptoms. There are also neutral and positive interpretations that won't be so taxing on your mental health!

- Hormone Therapy

Naturally, more estrogen means that more dopamine and serotonin are produced, helping to reverse and alleviate negative mental health issues.

- Practice self-care

Scientists have found that spending time in nature boosts your mood and self-esteem. It seems humans just really love nature. I mean, who doesn't love to watch a good sunset? Or gently watch the clouds float by in a clear, blue sky? Nature uplifts our mood and makes us feel much better. When driving to work, I often drive past a few farms with some cows grazing. Without fail, I glance at the cows every time (while keeping one eye on the road of course). They are just so peaceful, so fuzzy, and so cute! I may, or may not, have slowed my car down to moo at them a few times. Thankfully, there are no cameras around the fields. If there are, I maintain that that was not me in the video! I would also like to speak to a lawyer.

As we've already discussed in this chapter, another way to practice self-care is through exercise. Perimenopausal and menopausal women who exercise show fewer symptoms of depression than women who do not. If you are an avid runner or you workout regularly, you will already know that exercise boosts your mood. Scientifically, this is caused by the release of feel-good hormones like serotonin and dopamine. As agreed upon earlier, use exercise to legally get high. Soon, you'll get so addicted to that feeling of ecstasy that you won't ever want to miss an exercise session.

This, of course, does wonders for your body and your health, promoting good body image and all-round health, two factors that tend to improve people's mental health too. See how it's all a cycle?

There are so many other ways to practice self-care that the world is your oyster. The way you practice self-care should be particular to you. That means you need to find things that naturally make you relax and feel as though you've put all the weight on your shoulders away. Some people love fishing because the quiet allows them to meditate. Some people love yoga because the stretches allow them to release trapped emotions. Others love baking because the routine allows them to pause and rest their mind. Others love dancing because they can be free, let loose, and express their deepest emotions and thoughts without even speaking. Self-care is anything that you can do that is not typically harmful; that also allows you to care for your inner-most self and give your deepest parts of yourself a chance to breathe and to be cared for.

Additionally, make sleep an important part of your self-care. It is recommended that adults aged 26-64 years old get 7-9 hours of sleep each night. That means no more getting up at 2:00 a.m. to bury mustaches you shaved off in the middle of the night after sedating your husband. Perhaps I need to stop watching so many true crime shows, but the point still stands. Sleep, sleep, sleep!

You may also supplement your diet to get important nutrients and hormones (like serotonin and melatonin) that your body needs. Your doctor can test you for deficiencies and determine if supplements are a good idea for you.

- Seek support

We all need people to throw donuts at our heads when we're falling into that dark pit. We all stumble into that pit once in a while, but with understanding and compassionate family and friends, we can eventually find our way out. Keep in mind that spending time with people we love naturally releases dopamine, the anti-depression hormone.

Another way to seek support is to try to find support groups in your area or even online. You can try to find support groups for people going through tough times in their life, for people going through depression or for people going through menopause. Your doctor might be able to recommend some support groups. Alternatively, your doctor might be able to recommend you to a mental health specialist who is trained to help people dealing with mental health issues.

• Think positively

No matter how you might feel at the moment, it's good to remind yourself that menopause is a natural part of life. It is something all women go through. Even though you may be going through the worst of it now, it is not the end of everything. *This, too, shall pass!* Repeat this mantra on the days when menopause gets the best of your mental health.

Try to practice gratitude on a regular basis. Taking time to be grateful for all you have is a wonderful exercise for ushering in good feelings and happiness. Positive thinking and practicing gratitude are more powerful than you may realize. According to Dr. Lisa R. Yanek, Assistant Professor of Medicine at Johns Hopkins University, "People with a family history of heart disease who also had a positive outlook were one-third less likely to have a heart attack or other cardiovascular event within five to 25 years than those with a more negative outlook." Another study showed that thinking positively (and using deep breathing exercises) can improve feelings of restfulness and reduce feelings of worry, anxiety, and distress. Positive thinking also reduces long-term stress, which is known to destroy your immune system, leaving you more prone to developing mental health issues.

- Antidepressants

For some women going through menopause, holistic changes are enough to improve their mental health. For other women, this is not enough. Firstly, neither option is right or wrong. The only thing that's right is what is right for you. Secondly, if holistic options are not working, you can speak with your doctor about antidepressants. Antidepressants are medicines that treat the symptoms of depression, anxiety disorders, panic disorders, chronic pain, insomnia and even migraines.

Antidepressants work by increasing the level of neurotransmitters in your brain, including the level of serotonin in your brain. They are sometimes prescribed to reduce the symptoms of hot flashes and night sweats. For women who get intense hot flashes, alleviating this symptom can bring much needed stress relief, prompting good mental health.

Your doctor will very likely prescribe you the mildest antidepressant, known as Selective serotonin reuptake inhibitors (SSRIs). However, antidepressants come with side effects like all other medicines, including insomnia, nervousness, restlessness, nausea, dry mouth, and sexual problems. Your doctor will work with you to find the best type and dosage of antidepressant to provide you with the maximum benefit and the fewest side effects.

Menopause is as natural as dancing, childbirth, saying you don't want any fries, but then still asking to eat your partner's fries because they look so good and you didn't think they would smell so sexy, and the fresh scent of a baby after a bath. It is life.

The more accepting you are of this natural part of life, the more you can mentally brace yourself for it. At the same time, you can do everything right and still need additional support because of changing hormone and neurotransmitter levels in your body. This is also natural. With advances in medicine and psychology today, options exist to treat severe mental side effects of menopause. All this to say, you've got this!

With your mind at rest about the mental health side, let's explore other effects of menopause on the body, such as menopause's effects on your eyes, ears, heart function, sex life, and aches and pain. That's right. Just when you thought menopause couldn't possibly affect your life anymore, she comes back out for an *encore*. That's OK though, because you now have the mental resources to fight back. She clearly doesn't know you're prepared for this!

5

HOW TO STAY IN TOP PHYSICAL HEALTH

Despite advances in science, menopause seems to be a relatively uncharted field in medicine. It seems as though doctors just forgot that it exists. Or, more than likely, because women have simply put up with painful symptoms without so much as an "ouch," society has just assumed that we are comfortable where we are and don't need help.

As women get braver, and as we speak up about our symptoms, seeking treatment options, society be damned, the scientific field has to take it seriously. We're no longer just shutting up and putting up with it. Girl power! Or, to keep it real, woman power!

My favorite example of women speaking up happened in 2021 when British TV presenter Davina McCall (famous for presenting Big Brother UKr) released a documentary titled, *Sex, Myths and the Menopause,* where she explored menopause with refreshing honesty. Included in her documentary was criticism against the British medical community which had dismissed women's pressing medical needs for decades. Her boldness was refreshing and gave women the strength they needed to speak out about their experiences too. #davinamenopause trended on Twitter immediately following the documentary and Marie Claire UK reported that "the documentary was watched by more than two million people and resulted in 22,000 GPs [general practitioners] and nurses volunteering to complete a six-hour menopause course, while the demand for hormone replacement therapy (HRT) products surged by 30%."

She said about menopause: "Nobody told me about it. I hadn't learned about it at school, from my mum or my big sister. It was the thing nobody talked about. There was so much shame about it. It was a sign you'd dried up, you were past your sell-by date, you were at the end of your life, which in Victorian days, I suppose you were... but now we live until we're 80, we're right in the middle of our lives."

To empower you to live the second half of your life with the grace, sexiness, power, energy, and dynamism of a modern woman, this chapter will focus on how to stay in top physical health. You will have noticed a new crop of postmenopausal women in the media just killing it. From Angela Bassett (who must have a secret magic beauty well hidden in her backyard because there is no other explanation for her continued radiance and beauty) to the ever-classy, elegant Michele Obama, whose sexy outfits remind us we can continue to unleash our inner vixens whenever we choose no matter how old we are, to glowing-dewy-skin Helen Mirren, to the fitness pioneer, rock-hard-abs-boasting Davina McCall. These women are all proof that life and wellness after menopause is a very achievable reality.

Since we don't all have our own secret magic well like Mrs. Bassett, this chapter will explore the various ways in which you can maintain heart health, manage aches and pains during menopause, and keep your ears and eyes healthy during this time so you can achieve radiance from the inside out. It will also teach you how to maintain a healthy and enjoyable sex life during menopause. Let's start with the fun part!

SEX - KEEP THE FIRE BURNING!

Sex is nice. And while we're not all out here having sex like porn stars - or maybe you are and are really kinky in the bedroom, in which case, good for you - it's still nice to share intimate moments with your partner (or partners). The problem is that the menopausal drop in estrogen, progesterone, and testosterone can reduce your libido. Then there is the problem of having dry and thinning vaginal walls that can cause sex to be painful or uncomfortable. During menopause, blood flow to the lower vagina also decreases, which can cause a decrease in the sensations you feel during sex. Postmenopausal women can sometimes also experience a less sensitive clitoris. As with everything menopause, there is a wide range of symptoms you can experience, making things more complicated than it has to be. It is no surprise that 23% of women aged 57 to 85 do not find sex pleasurable. Despite this, only 3% of post-menopausal women report a noticeable loss in libido, meaning that most menopausal and postmenopausal women still love to get busy in the bedroom.

If very few women experience a change in libido, then the issue might not be menopause's physical symptoms as much as it is the effects these symptoms have on your relationship with sex. Changes in your body and even mind can cause you to feel uncomfortable in your body in general, especially if you are gaining weight, feel like you are losing the luster in your skin, and are developing dark undereye circles because night sweats keep you up all night. Since sex is very much physical, by following the guidance in various chapters of this book, you can reverse or improve many of these bodily changes so you can continue to feel like your regular old kinky self. Then again, sex is also as much physical as it is mental, which is why there is a lot of advice in this book on how to overcome the mental challenges of menopause.

If you are one of the 23% of women who don't find sex pleasurable, or if you are experiencing any other problems with sex and don't feel like dealing with the root cause, that is perfectly fine. Some women enjoy the newfound freedom gained from not pursuing sex. You have more time for yourself and more mental, emotional, and physical energy to pursue other interests in your life. No more feeling like a horny teenager just because a man who looks like George Clooney or Idris Elba walked in. If, on the other hand, you enjoy sex too much and would like to continue to salivate over sexy men, speak with your doctor about using hormone therapy to reverse some of the changes causing unpleasant sex.

Other methods for rekindling the fire include:

• Addressing discomfort

If you are feeling discomfort during sex, there is usually an underlying reason, such as changes in your vaginal wall or medications causing changes in your body.

Speak with your doctor about how to treat these changes. You may need to get off non-menopausal medications, pelvic surgery, or hormone therapy.

- Get tested

Since menopause covers such a large variety of symptoms, it is easy to mistake your symptoms for something else. Get tested regularly to rule out STDs as the cause of your symptoms. Plus, menopause does not give you the right to spread STDs all over willy-nilly, so get tested regularly!

- Explore different methods of intimacy

Penetrative sex is not the only form of sex you can enjoy. There are many other ways of enjoying intimacy with your partner(s), such as:

- Oral sex
- Explicit conversations or games
- Erotic massage

The National Women's Health Network advises: "Regular sex, either with a partner, through masturbation, or a combination of the two, definitely helps keep vaginal tissues more supple and moist. Extended sex play before insertion is always helpful, even if discomfort isn't severe. Liberal use of a water-soluble lubricant is often enough to make intercourse more comfortable."

• Communicate with your partner

As with premenopausal sex, menopausal and post-menopausal sex relies on good communication with your partner. Good sex is built on good communication (and a sturdy mattress).

• Kegel exercises

Do me a favor, and don't type "kegel sex" into the search bar when searching for kegel exercises to do to improve sex. Well, do search for it if you are looking for some *untraditional* videos to spice up the bedroom with your partner (or partners). If you want to look up kegel exercises, it might be best to use more specific terms if you want to avoid scarring yourself psychologically with some of the search options on the internet.

Kegels work by improving blood flow to the pelvic area, including the vagina. This improves arousal and lubrication, improving many menopausal symptoms related to sex.

WHAT'S WITH THE ACHES AND PAINS?

By now, you get the drill. I can't believe menopause is so bad, and I can't believe there are even more symptoms after all we've discussed in this book. I'm sorry to confirm it, but there are. Joint pain, fatigue, aches, and foot pain are typical menopausal symptoms. But what causes them?

Estrogen plays an important role in your body's calcium absorption. Without estrogen, many menopausal women develop osteoarthritis and osteoporosis. It is also common for menopausal women to develop rheumatoid arthritis, an autoimmune disease. Osteoarthritis and osteoporosis wreak havoc on your joints and bones. Rheumatoid arthritis, on the other hand, is an autoimmune disease that causes your immune system to attack the cells around your joints. This leads to swollen, painful, and stiff joints.

The Effect of Hormone Changes on Muscles, Joints, and Pain

Some of the effects of hormone changes on muscles, joints, and pain include:

- Migraine headaches

You may have noticed that you are more apt to develop headaches and migraines before or during your period. That's because migraines can be caused by hormonal changes in your body. Both estrogen and progesterone affect chemicals in the brain that cause headaches and migraines. Hence, the decline of both hormones can lead to constant migraines, particularly for women in perimenopause, when hormone levels fall at their steepest.

- Bruising

Don't be shocked if you wake up some mornings with unexplained bruises on your body or if every little bump causes bruises. Your skin becomes more prone to bruises during menopause as a result of lower estrogen levels. This decline causes the level of the protein collagen in your skin to fall (as we'll discuss more in Chapter Eight). Collagen is what makes your skin look plump and full, giving you that youthful look. With lower collagen levels, your skin gets thinner, becoming easily bruised.

Additionally, our fat tissues naturally thin out as we age, and our blood vessels lose elasticity. This makes them more likely to break, causing bruises. If you are on certain medications, like anticoagulants, corticosteroids, and non-steroidal anti-inflammatory drugs, this also increases your risk of bruising.

I advise you to stock up on foundation for your skin tone so you don't have to go out with people concerned that you may have a bully beating you up for your lunch

134 | ELLA RENÉE

money. Apply sunscreen consistently to prevent your skin from thinning out further. Make sure it is at least SPF 30. Ice packs applied for 15 minutes as soon as the bruise develops work wonders. You can also improve the efficiency of ice packs by applying a heated pad or warm cloth to the area after 48 hours.

You can tackle the root cause of the condition by trying to balance out your hormones, either through natural means detailed in this book or through hormone therapy.

- Fibromyalgia

Fibromyalgia is a health disorder that is characterized by musculoskeletal pain. This is accompanied by memory issues, mood issues, sleep problems, and fatigue. The majority of sufferers of this condition are menopausal women between the ages of 40 and 55, although postmenopausal women tend to suffer the most severe symptoms. The connection between fibromyalgia, menopause, and estrogen still needs further study, but it is known that it is caused by a decline in estrogen levels in the body. Unfortunately, hormone therapy is not an effective treatment for this, although estrogen patches seem to bring mild improvement. If you notice any of the symptoms of fibromyalgia, speak to your doctor about treatment options.

HEART HEALTH DURING MENOPAUSE

Menopause is infamous for its effects on heart health since it increases your risk of developing heart disease. Yes, the main culprit, once again, is estrogen. Scientists believe that estrogen has a positive effect on the outer lining of your heart's artery wall. This makes it easier for blood to flow through your heart. Restricted blood flow to and from your heart increases your risk of developing cardiovascular disease. Currently, scientists do not recommend hormone therapy to reduce your risk of developing cardiovascular disease. In fact, hormone therapy increases the risk of blood clots and strokes in older women. Naturally, eating healthy and exercising regularly will reduce your risk of developing heart disease.

Other ways in which hormonal changes in menopause affect health include:

- Your blood vessels may become stiffer
- Your risk of developing high blood pressure increases
- Your LDL, i.e., cholesterol levels may increase
- Your triglycerides (fat) levels may increase
- Your blood sugar levels may increase
- Your lean muscle mass may decrease

Women who are at risk of developing heart disease at menopause include:

- Women who have diabetes
- Women who smoke
- Women who have high blood pressure
- Women with high LDL, i.e., bad cholesterol
- Women with low HDL, i.e., good cholesterol
- Obese women
- Women with inactive lifestyles
- Women with a family history of heart disease

Heart Palpitations

When you have heart palpitations, your heart feels as though it's racing and skipping. Some women describe it as your heart feeling as though it's flipping or fluttering. Heart palpitations occur when your heart rate suddenly slows down, speeds up, or begins beating irregularly. You will feel it in your neck or chest or even both areas together. They occur in tandem with hot flashes, causing anxiety. This anxiety, ironically, then causes your heart to beat even faster.

Heart palpitations are caused by hormonal changes and are triggered by stress, sugar, and carb consumption, as well as overexertion through physical fitness, exercise, or sex (wink wink!). Seriously though, if you get heart palpitations during sex, stop being such a cougar and tone it down!

Heart palpitations typically last a few seconds. Nonetheless, if you experience them, you should see your doctor to ensure your symptoms are not caused by more serious conditions. I'll be the first to admit that there are times I treat my health like I treat my check engine light. If my car has not broken down, exploded, and turned to dust, then it is just flashing the check engine light for attention, and there clearly is nothing to check. It's not very healthy or wise, but we all do it, so don't dare judge me! If your palpitations increase in regularity or severity or if they begin to last more than a few minutes, accompanied by increased heart rate and weakness, then this is a sign that your body's "check heart" sign is blinking furiously. See a doctor!

As well as heart palpitation, possible symptoms of heart disease in women include:

- Nausea
- Vomiting
- Shortness of breath
- Chest pain
- Fatigue
- Swelling in your feet or ankles

You can reduce your risk of heart disease during menopause by:

- Telling your doctor about any irregular heartbeats
- Avoiding smoking
- Watching your weight
- Using supplements
- Exercising regularly
- Following a healthy diet
- Controlling other medical conditions by following your doctor's advice and treatment plan

EYE HEALTH DURING MENOPAUSE

Another common concern of menopause is how it affects eye health. I used to have a client, Mary, who would carry a small bottle of eye drops with her around the gym, stopping our sessions periodically to use them. Eventually, I began adding eye drop breaks to her workout routine so she could relieve her dry eyes.

We don't need to go into hormonal changes again. It's like making bread. There are so many different methods and ingredients, but the basic methodology is the same. In this case, the type of bread menopause is baking is dry eyes.

Symptoms of dry eyes include:

- Blurry vision
- Red eyes
- Burning eye pain
- Vision that comes and goes

An optician will be able to check that everything is OK with your eyes, menopause symptoms notwithstanding. They will also check for glaucoma and cataracts because your risk of developing both increases with menopause.

Treatment options for dry eyes include:

- Staying hydrated
- Eating healthy
- Eye drops without preservatives
- Lubricating ointments and gels
- Prescription medications
- Using a humidifier
- Limiting screen time
- Avoiding contact lenses

Treatment options for glaucoma include:

- Medication
- Eye drops

- Surgery
- Laser treatment

Treatment options for cataracts include:

- Surgery

EAR HEALTH DURING MENOPAUSE

Surprisingly, menopause can also affect your ears. As your estrogen level falls, the mucus membranes in your inner ears dry out. This leads to common ear problems, like:

- Hearing loss
- Painful ears
- Blocked ears
- Tinnitus (ringing in ears)
- Loss of balance/Dizziness

Treatment options include:

- Staying well-hydrated
- Eating healthily
- Using sea buckthorn oil supplements
- Changing medication

- Reducing your consumption of caffeine, high salt, and high sugar food

Estrogen. Estrogen. Estrogen. That one hormone seems to have just changed everything in your life. You used to be untouchable, and now, you have to worry about getting blocked ears or making sure you didn't leave your eye drops at home on your way to your lover's house for some kegel sex. I told you not to watch those videos, but since you chose to do so, I hope for your sake that your partner has a sturdy mattress.

6

EXERCISE FOR WEIGHT LOSS

F inally, after so much emphasis on exercise in previous chapters, we have reached the actual exercise component. In this chapter, we will look at the best types of exercise for weight loss and to strengthen your heart in the process.

In general, women tend to want to lose weight more than men. According to the CDC (Centers for Disease Control and Prevention), a higher percentage of women (56.4%) than men (41.7%) have tried to lose weight. I don't think we needed the CDC to tell us that, although it's nice to have official confirmation. This makes sense because our bodies carry more fat than men, we tend to gain weight more easily than men because of things like pregnancy and menopause, and there is just a general societal pressure on us to have low body fat at all times.

Before we move on in this chapter, I want to reiterate that losing weight is a self-love journey. You lose weight because you want to reduce your likelihood of developing serious health conditions like diabetes. You lose weight because perhaps you don't like how you look when overweight. You lose weight to reduce the amount of medication you need to stay healthy. You lose weight so you can be around for a long time to spend time with your kids and grandkids. These are all happy reasons to lose weight.

Conversely, you do not try to lose weight because you feel societal pressure on you to be perfect. Of course, this is much easier said than done because any woman knows how judgemental society is of women's bodies. And it's quite unfortunate because it's not just men judging our bodies constantly. It seems to be other women who judge and criticize our bodies even more. It's easy to get swept up in that fervor and want to lose weight to prove something to others. If you feel that you have an unhealthy relationship with your weight, it may be worth seeing a therapist to help you along in your weight loss journey so that it does not become a journey of self-hate, or one where you are desperately seeking validation from people who don't even care about you.

In general, I can classify my clients into two different sets of people: the women who are losing weight out of self-love and love for their families, and the women who are trying to lose weight because they feel it would win the love and validation of the outside world. The former set of women are usually happy, disciplined, and focused, even if they do sneak eat food on the "no-no" list once in a while, thinking I won't be able to tell. Protip: If you have a personal trainer, they can tell when you ate that slab of chocolate cake you said you didn't. Don't think lying will work, your body gives you away every time!

The latter set of women, on the other hand, tend to be miserable and so overfocused, they want to push themselves past the point of what is healthy. I don't need to tell you what set of women is the healthier, less stressed out, happier version.

"FAT" – THE UNINVITED GUEST: WHY WOMEN GAIN WEIGHT AT MENOPAUSE

There are five main reasons why women gain weight during menopause:

- Loss of muscle mass

Another function estrogen is responsible for is our muscle mass, i.e., lean muscle mass. If you don't know what lean muscle mass is, think of those biology pictures that you see in your doctor's office that show the inner parts of the human body. The red meaty parts that look like beef are your muscle mass. Muscle burns more calories at rest, so a decrease in muscle mass means that you need fewer calories than you did pre-menopause. If you're not able to appropriately decipher how much fewer calories you need, this can quickly lead to weight gain.

- Estrogen levels drop

Your hormonal levels play an important role in your distribution of body fat. For instance, some men who gain a lot of weight see an increase in estrogen, which then causes them to develop breasts. Too much estrogen increases fat storage, but so does too little. Essentially, your body is just high maintenance and demands the exact hormonal balance, or it will throw a tantrum.

- Other aging-related issues

Honestly, sometimes you just want to sit on the couch, eat a cookie and catch up on your favorite TV show. In general, humans do tend to be lazy. So, as we enter middle age and start to get tired, we are less inclined to want to spend 20 minutes on the Stairmaster when we can be comfortable on the couch, resting. You specifically bought that couch because it was comfy, and now you're supposed to leave its beautiful warm embrace to almost die on a Stairmaster while stopping to use eye drops? Who thought up this brilliant idea?

To make it even less enticing, you have to workout for longer and at higher intensities than you did when you were a young spring chicken because your metabolism has slowed down (because of, you guessed it, changes in your hormone levels). Suddenly, the couch seems much more sexy! Maybe you'll even open that party-size bag of cookies to go with it!

- A less active lifestyle

Our lifestyles tend to become less active as we age naturally. Your kids grow up and move out, so you don't have to run after kids anymore. You are most likely more established in your career, meaning you're sat down for most of the day in a well-air-conditioned room or, in the colder months, in a room that's the perfect warm temperature for happiness. This is very different from your college years when you may have had to run for the bus a few times a week, do your own moving because you were too broke to afford movers, and lived in a dingy apartment that was too hot in the summer and too cold in the winter. It turns out not being financially established increases our metabolism. Middle age does bring more comfort and security in life, but too much comfort also leads to weight gain.

- Change in sleeping habits

Even without the added baggage of menopause, our sleeping patterns tend to naturally change as we age. This can be attributed to general hormonal changes related to aging but also because of changes in our life-style. If you spend the whole day on your feet working as a waitress to pay for college tuition, you probably start nodding off even before you get home from a long day.

On the other end of the spectrum, middle age is also a time when people see huge life changes, such as family members becoming deceased, kids moving out, divorces, retirement, and so on. All these changes, in conjunction with the hormonal tornado that is menopause, can leave you too stressed and anxious to really enjoy good sleep. Without regular good sleep, it is impossible to have the energy to exercise, causing you to gain weight.

BEST EXERCISES FOR WEIGHT LOSS AT 50 AND BEYOND

These exercises are the best exercise for weight loss for over-50s:

• Cardio

Cardio is great for weight loss because it's an aerobic exercise. Aerobic exercises promote weight loss because they burn calories. Burning calories is good because your body then has no extra calories to turn into fat. Cardio also increases your heart rate, giving your heart a good workout, strengthening your heart muscles, and keeping your arteries free of blockages. Furthermore, it promotes fat burning (especially when combined with regular strength training exercises).

Cardio exercises can be high-impact or low-impact. High impact means you make more impact on your joints when your feet hit the ground. Examples of high-impact exercises are running and skipping. High-impact exercises burn more calories because jumping and moving around with more impact burns more calories. That's why you can burn more calories running than walking in the same amount of time. Low-impact exercises are the opposite of high-impact exercises because they have little impact on your joints and feet. Some low-impact exercises, like swimming, can actually improve joint pain. In fact, don't let the name fool you. Some low-impact exercises, like cycling and swimming can seriously burn calories and increase your heart rate, especially when you do them consistently.

Some cardio exercises you can incorporate into your workout routine include:

- Swimming
- Cycling
- Running
- Walking
- HIIT (High-Intensity-Interval-Training)
- Stairmaster workouts (which are great for a tight, perky butt)

- Yoga

Yoga may not necessarily directly promote weight loss, but it is a great practice to improve your quality of sleep, especially as a menopausal woman. Good quality sleep allows your muscles to repair themselves and grow after a workout. Increased muscle mass speeds up your metabolism and gives you the strength and brute force you need to exercise more. Plus, yoga keeps your muscles and joints healthy and flexible, allowing you to do a full range of exercises and sexercises without any mobility issues.

• Pelvic floor exercises

Pelvic floor exercises (i.e., kegels) strengthen your pelvic region and promote blood flow to the area. This improves symptoms of menopause, such as incontinence, getting up frequently at night to urinate, bowel leaks, vaginal pain, and dry vaginal walls.

• Breathwork

Breathwork exercises help to relieve stress and promote relaxation. This eases menopausal symptoms like sleeplessness, mood swings, and anxiety. Some exercises, like yoga and mindfulness meditation, incorporate breathwork exercises in their practice.

• Mind-body activities

Mind-body activities, like yoga, tai chi, and mindfulness meditation, promote an internal search of your mind while sending breath to all areas of your body. By searching your mind, you bring to the forefront of your consciousness things that might be bothering you and causing stress and anxiety. You work through them, eliminating your bad mood in the process.

In some cases, mind-body exercises also incorporate stretching to promote the release of stress and other trapped negative emotions in various parts of your body. Some mind-body activities, like mindfulness meditation, can also be done while exercising.

- Strength training for weight loss

Strength training involves working out your muscles regularly. The goal is to increase your strength by steadily increasing the amount of weights you lift. Strength training increases muscle mass, which, in turn, increases your resting metabolic rate, slowing down the rate at which your body accumulates fat.

Try these strength training exercises and turn your body into a fat-burning machine:

Squats

1. Start by standing with your feet shoulder-width apart, toes pointing forward.
2. Keep your chest up and core engaged as you begin to lower your body down by bending your knees and pushing your hips back. Keep your weight on your heels, and make sure your

knees do not extend past your toes. Option to hold a dumbbell in hands.

3. Lower your body until your thighs are parallel to the ground, then push up through your heels to return to the starting position.

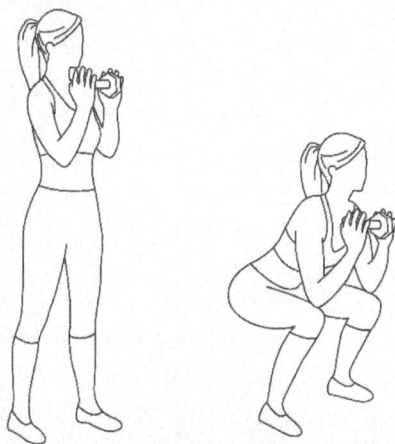

Chest press

1. Lie flat on the floor or a bench with your feet firmly planted on the ground. Hold the dumbbells at chest level with your palms facing forward.

2. Slowly lower the weights down towards your chest, keeping your elbows at a 90-degree angle.

3. Pause for a second, then push the weights back up to the starting position. Make sure to breathe steadily throughout the exercise and keep your core engaged.

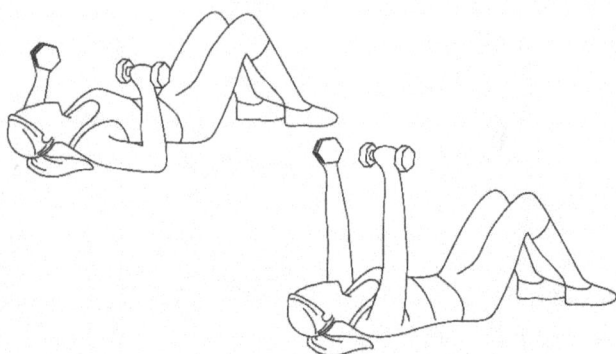

Stationary Lunges

1. Start by standing up straight with your feet shoulder-width apart. Then, take a big step back with one foot.
2. Bend both knees, bringing your back knee close to the ground. Both legs should also be bent at a 90-degree angle. Make sure your front knee doesn't go past your toes.
3. Hold this position for a second, then push back up to the starting position.

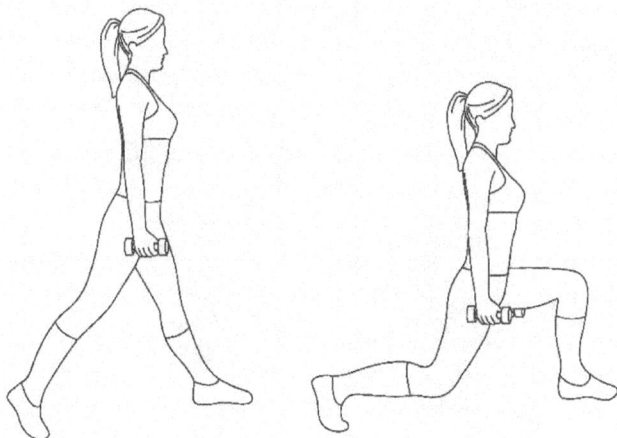

Deadlifts

1. Stand with your feet shoulder-width apart and hold a barbell or dumbbells with an overhand grip, making sure your hands are slightly wider than your shoulders.
2. Keep a slight bend in your knees, your back straight, and your core engaged. Slowly hinge from the hips lowering the weight just below your knees.
3. In a controlled manner, raise back up to the starting position.

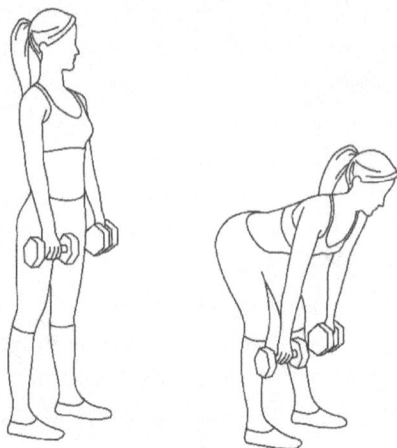

Dumbbell one-arm row

1. Start by standing with your feet shoulder-width apart and holding a dumbbell in one hand. Bend your knees and lean forward, keeping your back straight.
2. Pull the dumbbell up towards your chest, keeping your elbow close to your body and squeezing your shoulder blade at the top of the movement.
3. Lower the dumbbell back down and repeat reps before switching to the other arm. Remember to keep your core engaged and your breathing steady throughout the exercise.

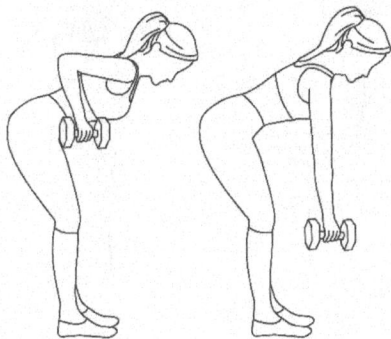

Dumbbell bicep curls

1. Start by standing straight with your feet shoulder-width apart and holding a dumbbell in each hand.
2. Keep your elbows close to your body and slowly lift the weights up towards your chest, bending at the elbow.
3. Pause for a second at the top of the movement, then slowly lower the weights back down to the starting position. Remember to keep your back straight and avoid swinging your arms to get the most out of this exercise.

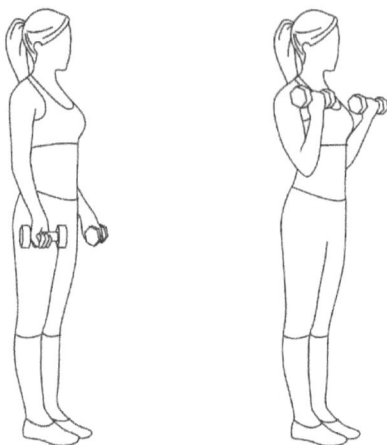

Plank

1. Lay face down on the floor, bend your arms and place your elbows in line with your shoulders. Point your toes down so that they are touching the floor.
2. Now raise your hips and chest off the floor. Your body should form a straight line from your head to your heels.
3. Engage your core muscles and hold this position for as long as you can. Remember to breathe evenly and to keep your hips level with the rest of your body. You can start by holding the plank for 30 seconds and gradually increase the time as you build up strength.

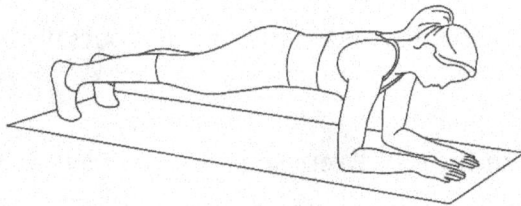

Now that you know how to perform the exercises, try following this simple workout routine. You can do this workout at home or in the gym. Remember to always start your workout with a 3-5 minute warmup. This can be anything from jumping jacks to a jog on the spot or my favorite, yup, you guessed it, burpees!

Complete 12-15 repetitions of each exercise and repeat each circuit three times.

A1: DeadliftsA2: Squats A3: Dumbbell one-arm row

B1: Lunges B2: Chest Press B3: Bicep curls

C1: Plank – Hold for as long as possible in proper positioning.

Once you've worked up a sweat and have finished your strength training session, be sure to stretch. Stretching after a workout is important to increase flexibility and reduce the risk of injury. It also helps to prevent muscle soreness and stiffness. Aim to target the major muscle groups worked. Remember to hold each stretch for at least 30 seconds and never push yourself past your limit.

There you have it. Exercise is a great way to defeat the evils of menopause, reverse negative symptoms and look good in the process. Not exercising is kind of like being offered a winning lottery ticket with no strings attached and refusing the offer. It's just not very smart.

7

WEIGHT LOSS WITH SIMPLE NUTRITION

Yes, you can lose weight even during perimenopause and menopause. Yes, lower estrogen levels make it more challenging to lose weight, but menopause does not know who she's messing with if she thinks you'll just let it go and give up without a fight.

In my line of work, about 50% of my clients are women in varying stages of menopause, training and eating healthy to keep their bodies in great shape! In this chapter, I will be providing you with a number of tips for how to lose weight with the right diet. This chapter also concludes with a lovingly hand-crafted, wonder-fully-curated, daintily-typed 28-day meal plan. But I don't want to oversell it.

NUTRITION AND DIET TIPS

You don't put just any kind of fuel in your car, so why would you put anything but the best in your body? Eating healthy foods is the best way to show your body how much you appreciate it for all it does for you, like allowing you to enjoy kegel sex or keeping you alive to watch unconventional videos of kegel sex.

When you eat right, you have more energy, more nutrients, and your body needs more time to digest your food. This allows you to increase the time between meals at the same time as it reduces your desire for unhealthy food. Ultimately, eating right makes weight loss possible.

Before we delve into the 28-day meal plan, let's briefly discuss some nutrition and diet tips for menopausal women, to better prepare you for this epic meal plan. These tips will give you a general idea of why I chose the meals and ingredients that I did in my meal plan.

Tip 1

Once puberty hits and women begin experiencing hormonal changes associated with menstrual cycles, pregnancy, childbearing, and menopause, we tend to need a lot more iron and folate because our risk of developing anemia increases. Women of childbearing age need twice as much iron as men because of the amount of blood they lose on a monthly basis. An iron-rich diet also prevents the development of mood disorders like depression. In addition, iron also promotes healthy skin, hair, and nails, so it is a lesser-known beauty secret.

Tip 2

Supplements are not enough. The clue is in the name. They supplement for occasional times when you don't get enough of a particular vitamin or mineral, but they are not solid replacements for getting nutrients from food. Eat a balanced diet to get a well-balanced amount of vitamins and minerals from food.

Tip 3

You need plenty of calcium in your diet to prevent depression, irritability, anxiety, and sleep difficulties. Calcium also keeps your teeth and bones strong. Eat calcium-rich foods in conjunction with magnesium and vitamin D-rich foods to allow for proper absorption of calcium. At the same time, women's risk of developing osteoporosis and weakened bones is greater than men's, which is why we also need more vitamin D, calcium, and magnesium in our diets.

Tip 4

Your saturated fat intake should be no more than 10% of your daily calorie intake.

Tip 5

Eat plenty of dietary fiber to ward off Type 2 diabetes.

Tip 6

Swap salt for other seasonings, like onion powder, paprika, citrus fruits, and fresh herbs. Salt leads to high blood pressure, particularly in women over the age of 50.

Tip 7

Watch how many calories you consume. Even consuming 100 calories over your Recommended Daily Allowance (RDA) each day will lead to weight gain over a short period of time. It is not recommended for menopausal women to be overweight or obese because it severely increases their risk of developing health conditions like diabetes.

Tip 8

Eat prebiotic and probiotic-rich foods. Probiotic-rich foods will increase the amount of good bacteria in your digestive system, while prebiotic-rich foods will improve your calcium absorption.

Tip 9

Eat plenty of fruits and vegetables with each meal. In fact, half of your plate at every meal should be fruits and vegetables. This boosts your immune system and reduces inflammation. Inflammation is a main culprit in the development of serious health conditions like diabetes, heart disease, and cancer.

FOODS TO AVOID IN A WEIGHT LOSS MEAL PLAN

Foods to avoid in a weight loss meal plan are:

- Sugary foods

Sugar offers a great way to gain weight in no time, whilst increasing your risk of developing various health conditions, including tooth-related problems, diabetes, and heart disease. Sure, cake and cookies taste really good, but sugar comes at a steep cost! It's a shame that something that tastes so good wants to kill us. Imagine if sugar had the same effect on our bodies as eating a bowl of spinach and kale salad. You could eat chocolate cake all day and still lose weight and be healthy. That sounds like the perfect dream.

- Alcohol

Alcohol contains a huge amount of empty calories that only speed up weight gain whilst also causing inflammation. It comes with a host of negative health effects and is best left alone.

- Salty foods

Sodium causes you to retain water in your body, causing what is known as water weight (looking and feeling bloated) and unwanted weight gain.

28-DAY RECIPES & MEAL PLAN

How often do you say to yourself, "I should really start eating better," well, you're in the right place. Don't worry, I'm not going to force-feed you kale smoothies all day or make you count the individual grains of brown rice in your bowl. I'm here to make healthy eating as painless as possible with my 28-day meal plan. And the best part is that you get to take control by choosing the meals you find most drool-worthy. Choose from the selection of breakfast, lunch, and dinner options to create your own desired meal plan, or follow my daily recommendations at the end of the recipes.

Quick tip: Save time and meal prep by doubling or tripling the portion sizes.

Breakfast Recipes

Almond Flour Pancakes

Servings: 1

<u>Ingredients</u>

- ¼ cup almond flour
- 1 tsp. baking powder
- 2 eggs
- ½ banana
- 1 tsp. coconut oil
- 1 tsp. maple syrup
- Handful of blueberries

<u>Directions</u>

In a food processor, blend flour, eggs, baking powder, banana, and coconut oil. Pour batter into a non-stick pan, turning pancakes over when bubbles form. Cook for an additional two minutes. Dress them with maple syrup and blueberries.

Nutritional Information

Calories: 376 kcal, Fat: 18g, Carbs: 28g, Protein: 24, Sugars: 5g, Fiber:7g

Egg Muffin Bites

Serving size: 1

Ingredients

- 3 eggs
- 2-3 kale leaves
- 1 tomato
- 1 green pepper
- 1oz goat cheese
- 1/2 tsp. dried basil
- 1/2 tsp. salt

Directions

Cut veggies into small pieces. In one bowl, mix all ingredients together. Take 3 muffin molds and fill them up with the mixture. Bake them in the oven at 360°F/180°C for 20 minutes.

Nutritional Information

Calories: 280 kcal, Fat: 12g, Carbs: 6g, Protein: 21g, Sugars: 0, Fiber: 3g

Blueberry Oatmeal Bowl

Serving size: 1

Ingredients

- 1 cup oat milk
- 2 tsp. natural peanut butter
- ¼ cup oat flakes
- Handful of blueberries

Directions

In a pot add oat milk, peanut butter, half blueberries, and oat flakes. Cook them until boiling. When the mixture gets sticky you can serve your oatmeal. Top the oatmeal with the rest of the blueberries.

Nutritional Information

Calories: 388 kcal, Fat: 11 tsp., Carbs: 40g, Protein: 14g, Sugars: 1g, Fiber: 9g

Anti-Inflammatory Smoothie

Serving size: 1

Ingredients

- ½ cup frozen berries
- ¼ avocado
- 1 tsp. chia seeds
- ½ cup spinach leaves
- ⅔ cup kefir
- 2 tsp. almond butter

Directions

Place all ingredients in a blender and blend until smooth. Serve on ice.

Nutritional Information

Calories: 410 kcal, Fat: 20g, Carbs: 43g, Protein: 18g, Sugars: 2g, Fiber: 10g

Avocado Toast with Poached Eggs

Servings: 1

Ingredients

- 2 slices whole grain bread

- 2 eggs
- ½ avocado
- salt and pepper, to taste
- Herbs, to season
- Heirloom tomatoes, quartered (optional)

Directions

Boil water in a pot, using enough water to cover your eggs as they poach.

Turn off the heat once the water boils. Carefully crack two eggs into the pot of water. Cover the pot for 4-5 minutes. As the eggs cook, toast the bread and lay them flat on a plate. Smash the avocado and layer on each piece of toast. Lift the eggs out of the pot of hot water using a slotted cooking spoon, then place the eggs onto the avocado toast. Season with salt, pepper, and herbs. Serve with heirloom tomatoes, if desired.

Nutritional Information

Calories: 393 kcal, Fat: 17g, Carbs: 30g, Protein: 20g, Sugars: 1g, Fiber: 8g

Yogurt Fruit Bowl

Serving size: 1

Ingredients

- 1 cup Greek yogurt
- 2 tbsp almonds
- 2 tbsp granola
- ½ cup mixed berries

Directions

Mix the yogurt with almonds and granola. Top with fruit.

Nutritional Information

Calories: 375 kcal, Fat: 5g, Carbs: 29g, Protein: 21g, Sugars: 5g, Fiber: 8g

Apple Muffins

Serving size: 1

Ingredients

- 1 egg
- 1 small chopped apple
- 1 tsp coconut oil

- 3 tbsp. oat milk
- 1 tsp maple syrup
- 3 tbsp oat flakes
- 1 tsp baking powder
- Pinch of cinnamon

Directions

Place dry ingredients; oat flakes, baking powder, and cinnamon, in a bowl and mix together. In a separate bowl, mix all the wet ingredients, egg, milk, coconut oil, and maple syrup together. Stir the wet ingredients into the dry ingredients. Fold the chopped apple into the mixture. Take 2 muffin molds and fill them with the mixture. Bake in the oven at 400°F/204°C for 15-20 minutes.

Nutritional Information

Calories: 346 kcal, Fat: 6g, Carbs: 39g, Protein: 11g, Sugars: 5g, Fiber:11g

Overnight Kiwi and Chia

Serving size: 1

Ingredients

- 3 tbsp. chia seeds

- 1 tbsp. oat flakes
- 1 tbsp. natural peanut butter
- 1 tsp. maple syrup
- 1 cup oat or almond milk
- 1 kiwi

Directions

Mix together chia seeds, peanut butter, maple syrup and milk. Let sit overnight. Top with oats and kiwi.

Nutritional Information

Calories: 425 kcal, Fat:16g, Carbs:42g, Protein:13g, Sugars: 6g, Fiber: 10g

Detox Protein Smoothie

Serving size: 1

Ingredients

- ½ avocado
- 1 banana
- Handful of spinach
- 1 scoop vanilla protein powder
- ½ cup oat or almond milk

Directions

Cut up banana and avocado. Place all ingredients in a food processor and blend them until smooth.

Nutritional Information

Calories: 380 kcal, Fat: 14g, Carbs: 16g, Protein: 34g, Sugars: 2g, Fiber: 3g

Spinach Omelet

Serving size: 1

Ingredients

- 2 eggs
- 1 handful baby spinach
- 1/3 cup shredded mozzarella
- 1 cup cherry tomatoes
- 1 tsp. Olive oil
- Pinch of salt and pepper

Directions

In a preheated cooking pan, add olive oil and eggs. Scramble the eggs and mix them with salt and pepper. Cook for 2 minutes on medium heat, flip, and cook for 2 more minutes. Top with mozzarella and spinach—place cherry tomatoes on the side.

Nutritional Information

Calories: 320 kcal, Fat: 16g, Carbs: 9g, Protein: 26g, Sugars: 0g, Fiber: 1g

Yogurt Banana Split

Serving size: 1

Ingredients:

- 1 banana
- ½ cup blueberries
- ½ cup raspberries
- 1 cup low-fat Greek yogurt
- 2 tbsp. Granola

Directions

Slice the banana in half horizontally and separate on a plate. Put the yogurt in between the banana slices. Add berries and granola on top.

Nutritional Information

Calories: 370 kcal, Fat: 18g, Carbs: 23g, Protein: 22g, Sugars: 6g, Fiber: 6g

Pineapple Kale Smoothie

Serving size: 1

Ingredients

- 1 cup chopped pineapple
- Handful of kale
- 1 cup almond milk
- ½ tsp. Cinnamon
- 1 tsp. Natural peanut butter

Directions

Place all ingredients in a food processor and blend them until smooth. Serve on ice.

Nutritional Information

Calories: 323 kcal, Fat: 10g, Carbs: 22g, Protein: 7g, Sugars: 5g, Fiber: 4g

Lunch Recipes

Chicken Salad

Serving size: 1

<u>Ingredients</u>

- 1 medium chicken breast
- ½ avocado
- 1 handful lettuce
- ½ cucumber
- 5 cherry tomatoes
- Pinch of salt
- 1 tbsp. olive oil
- 1 tsp. vinegar

<u>Directions</u>

Grill the chicken for 10 minutes. Cut the veggies and place them in a bowl. Cut the chicken and mix it with the veggies. Dress your salad with olive oil, salt, and vinegar.

<u>Nutritional Information</u>

Calories: 410 kcal, Fat: 21g, Carbs: 8g, Protein: 28g, Sugars: 0g, Fiber: 4g

Quinoa Bowl

Serving size: 1

Ingredients

- ¾ raw quinoa
- ½ cup broccoli
- ¼ onion
- ¼ cup pomegranate
- 1 small chicken breast
- 1 tbsp. olive oil
- Little lemon juice
- Salt
- Pepper

Directions

Bake chicken breast in the oven at 350°F/177°C for 25 minutes. Boil quinoa for 15 minutes, drain, and place in a bowl together with broccoli flowers, chopped onion, and pomegranate. Cut chicken into cubes and add to the bowl. Dress all with olive oil, lemon juice, salt, and pepper.

Nutritional Information

Calories: 570, Fat: 21g, Carbs: 57g, Protein: 28g, Sugars: 3g, Fiber: 9g

Salmon and Spinach Salad

Serving size: 1

Ingredients

- 1 cup baby spinach
- Salmon fillet
- ¼ cup cherry tomatoes
- ½ avocado
- ¼ cucumber
- 1 tsp. olive oil
- 1 tsp. lemon juice
- ½ tsp. vinegar
- Salt

Directions

Place the spinach in a bowl, and add cherry tomatoes, avocado, cucumber, and salmon. Dress the salad with olive oil, lemon juice, salt, and vinegar.

Nutritional Information

Calories: 425 kcal, Fat: 31g, Carbs: 9g, Protein: 22g, Sugars: 0g, Fiber: 3g

Stuffed Pepper

Serving size: 1

Ingredients

- 1 bell pepper
- 2.5oz cooked ground beef
- ¼ cup cooked brown rice
- ½ cup tomato sauce
- ½ tsp. salt
- ½ tsp. pepper
- ½ tsp. paprika

Directions

Mix ground beef, spices, and rice. Cut open the top of the pepper and take the handle and seeds out. Fill the pepper with the mixture. Top with tomato sauce and bake it in the oven for 20 minutes at 400°F/204°C.

Nutritional Information

Calories: 476 kcal, Fat: 14g, Carbs: 26g, Protein: 31g, Sugars: 2g, Fiber: 2g

Mediterranean Veggie Wrap

Serving size: 1

Ingredients

- 1 whole wheat tortilla wrap
- 1 tbsp. hummus
- ¼ cup feta cheese
- ¼ onion
- ¼ cucumber
- ½ bell pepper

Directions

Spread the hummus on the wrap. Chop veggies and add to wrap with the cheese. Wrap it well and bake it in the oven for 10 minutes at 350°F/177°C.

Nutritional Information

Calories: 430 kcal, Fat: 14g, Carbs: 34g, Protein: 18g, Sugars: 2g, Fiber: 6g

Zucchini Pasta with Ground Beef

Serving size: 1

Ingredients

- 1 zucchini
- 3.5oz ground beef
- ½ cup tomato sauce
- ½ tsp. garlic powder
- Salt and pepper
- ¼ cup parmesan cheese
- 2 tsp. Olive oil

Directions

Cut the zucchini into thin, long stripes. Add ½ the oil on a cooking pan and place in the beef, spices, and salt. Fry it for 6 minutes, then add the tomato sauce, cover, and cook for 10 minutes. In a separate pan, add the other half of the olive oil and fry the zucchini for 10 minutes. Place zucchini on a plate and add the beef and tomato sauce. Serve the pasta with shredded parmesan.

Nutritional Information

Calories: 401 kcal, Fat: 18g, Carbs: 9g, Protein: 28g, Sugars: 3g, Fiber: 5g

Chicken Teriyaki and Salad

Serving size: 1

<u>Ingredients</u>

- 1 medium chicken breast
- ½ tsp. low-sodium teriyaki sauce
- Salt and pepper
- 1 tbsp. Olive oil
- 1 cup mixed greens
- 1 tbsp. Caesar dressing

<u>Directions</u>

Cut the chicken into strips. Place it on a cooking pan together with olive oil, teriyaki sauce, salt, and pepper. Stir fry for 10 minutes. Place mixed greens on a plate and add Caesar dressing. Put chicken strips on top.

<u>Nutritional Information</u>

Calories: 403 kcal, Fat: 13g, Carbs: 8g, Protein: 24g, Sugars: 2g, Fiber: 1g

Tabouli Salad

Serving size: 1

<u>Ingredients</u>

- ½ cup cooked quinoa
- ¼ cup olives
- ¼ cup feta cheese
- 1 tomato
- ¼ onion
- ½ tbsp. lemon juice
- 1 tsp. Olive oil
- ¼ cup parsley
- Pinch salt

<u>Directions</u>

Chop olives, tomato, onion and, parsley into small pieces and mix them in a bowl. Add the cooked quinoa, feta, salt, olive oil, and lemon juice. Mix well and serve.

<u>Nutritional Information</u>

Calories: 374 kcal, Fat: 17g, Carbs: 37g, Protein: 21g, Sugars: 1g, Fiber: 7g

Falafel Avocado Wrap with Garlic Aioli

Servings: 3

Ingredients

- 1 can chickpeas, drained
- 1 whole wheat wrap
- 3 tablespoons chickpea flour
- ½ avocado
- Handful of lettuce
- ½ tomato
- ½ cup onion
- ½ cup chopped parsley
- ½ cup fresh chopped cilantro
- 1 small habanero pepper, finely chopped
- 4 garlic cloves, finely chopped
- 1 teaspoon cumin
- 1 teaspoon salt
- ½ tsp cardamom
- ¼ teaspoon black pepper
- ½ teaspoon baking soda
- Olive oil for frying

Ingredients for the garlic aioli

- ½ cup low-fat mayonnaise (vegan preferred)
- 1 tablespoon lemon juice

- 1 clove garlic, minced
- 1 teaspoon extra virgin oil
- ⅓ teaspoon pepper

Directions

Add onion, herbs, chickpeas, salt, pepper, and black pepper into a food processor. Pulse until the mixture is coarse. In a large bowl, add the chickpea mixture, chickpea flour, and baking soda, then mix. Take the mixture out of the fridge, then make similar-sized falafel balls. Bake for 25-30 minutes at 375° F/190°C.

To make the garlic aioli, mix all the ingredients together.

Place falafel balls, lettuce, tomato, avocado, and garlic aioli in a whole wheat wrap.

Nutritional Information

Calories: 400 kcal, Fat: 10g, Carbs: 20g, Sugars: 5g, Protein: 7g, Fiber: 5g

Chicken and Veggie Skewers

Serving size: 1

<u>Ingredients</u>

- 3.5oz chicken
- 1 red pepper
- 1 yellow pepper
- ¼ onion
- ½ lemon
- Salt
- 1tbs. olive oil

<u>Directions</u>

Cut the chicken, peppers, and onion into squares. Assemble on the skewers. Preheat the grill and spread 1 tsp. olive oil on it. Bake each side of the skewers for 5-10 minutes.

<u>Nutritional Information</u>

Calories: 498 kcal, Fat: 16g, Carbs: 32g Protein: 31g, Sugars: 1g, Fiber: 8g

Spinach Frittata With Millet

Serving size: 1

<u>Ingredients</u>

- 1 cup spinach
- ½ cup cooked millet
- 3 eggs
- 1 tbsp. olive oil
- Salt and pepper

<u>Directions</u>

Preheat the oven to 375°F/190°C. Place oil in a small oven pot, mix spinach with millet, eggs, and salt and pepper. Bake it for 25 minutes.

<u>Nutritional Information</u>

Calories: 335 kcal, Fat: 19g, Carbs: 34g, Protein: 21g, Sugars: 1g, Fiber: 11g

Chicken Protein Soup

Serving size: 1

Ingredients

- 2.6oz chicken thighs
- ¼ cup quinoa
- 1 small carrot
- 2 cloves Garlic
- ¼ onion
- 2 cups low-sodium vegetable broth
- Cilantro

Directions

Boil all ingredients together for 30 minutes. At the end, take the chicken thighs and shred them in small pieces. Top with fresh cilantro.

Nutritional Information

Calories: 482 kcal, Fat: 17g, Carbs: 38g, Protein: 23g, Sugars: 1g, Fiber: 6g

Dinner Recipes

Chicken Stir Fry

Serving size: 1

Ingredients

- 1 chicken breast
- ½ cup broccoli
- ¼ cup mushrooms
- 1 red pepper
- 1 tbsp. olive oil
- 2 tsp. soy sauce
- 1 cup chicken broth

Directions

Add olive oil to stir fry pan and heat on medium. Cut the mushrooms, red pepper, broccoli, and chicken and add them to the pan. Stir fry them for 5 minutes, then pour in the broth and soy sauce. Cover the pan and cook for 15 minutes.

Nutritional Information

Calories: 423 kcal, Fat: 26g, Carbs: 25g, Protein: 28g, Sugars: 3g, Fiber: 6g

Salmon and Noodles

Serving size: 1

Ingredients

- 2 tsp. pesto
- 3.5oz salmon
- ½ cup uncooked rice noodles
- Salt and pepper
- Parmesan cheese

Directions

Bake the salmon in the oven for 15 minutes at 400°F/204°C. Boil noodles in a pot until soft. When the noodles are ready, drain and mix them with pesto sauce. Cut the salmon and place on top of the noodles. Top with salt, pepper, and parmesan cheese.

Nutritional Information

Calories: 460 kcal, Fat: 18g, Carbs: 41g, Protein: 26g, Sugars: 1g, Fiber: 1g

Chicken Fajitas

Serving size: 1

<u>Ingredients</u>

- 1 chicken breast
- ½ green pepper
- ½ red pepper
- ½ tomato
- ¼ onion
- ½ tsp. garlic powder
- ½ tsp. ground coriander
- 1 tbsp. salsa
- 1 tsp. olive oil
- ½ tsp. salt
- 1 whole wheat tortilla

<u>Directions</u>

Heat a cooking pan on medium heat and add the oil. Cut the veggies and chicken into small pieces. Place the veggies and chicken, and all spices into the pan and stir-fry them for 15 minutes. Add the fried mixture to a tortilla wrap. Top with salsa.

Nutritional Information

Calories: 416 kcal, Fat: 13g, Carbs: 38g, Protein: 27g, Sugars: 6g, Fiber: 3g

Chickpea Stew

Serving size: 1

Ingredients

- 1 cup canned chickpeas
- ¼ onion
- 1 tomato
- ½ red pepper
- 1 diced carrot
- ¼ tsp garlic powder
- ¼ tsp paprika
- 1 cup vegetable broth
- Pinch of salt
- 1 tbsp. Olive oil

Directions

Place all ingredients together in a cooking pot and let them simmer for 25 minutes.

Nutritional Information

Calories: 413 kcal, Fat: 28g, Carbs: 29g, Protein: 23g, Sugars: 1g, Fiber: 9g

Shrimp Dish with Veggies

Serving size: 1

Ingredients

- 4oz shrimp
- 5 asparagus sticks
- Handful of green beans
- ½ red pepper
- ¼ cup mushrooms
- 1 tbsp. Olive oil
- ½ tsp. paprika
- ½ tsp. Curry powder
- Salt and pepper

Directions

Cut all veggies into small pieces. In a non-stick pan, add olive oil and heat on medium heat. Add all ingredients to the pan and sauté for 15 minutes.

Nutritional Information

Calories: 357, Fat: 17g, Carbs: 43g, Protein: 33g, Sugars: 0g, Fiber: 8g

Taco Bowl

Serving size: 1

Ingredients

- 1 cup chopped romaine lettuce
- ½ cup ground beef cooked
- ½ bell pepper
- Handful cherry tomatoes
- 1 tbsp. chopped chili pepper
- ¼ cup scallions
- ¼ cup shredded cheese
- Taco seasoning

Directions

Precook the beef with the taco seasoning, then place in a bowl. Add all other ingredients on top.

Nutritional Information

Calories: 455 kcal, Fat: 17.5g, Carbs: 34g, Protein: 27g, Sugars: 3g, Fiber: 9g

Ground Turkey Chili

Serving size: 1

Ingredients

- 3 oz ground turkey
- ½ green pepper
- ½ red pepper
- ½ onion
- ¼ cup black beans
- 1 cup crushed tomatoes
- ¼ cup corn
- ½ tsp. Garlic powder
- Cilantro
- Salt and pepper

Directions

Precook the ground turkey and cut peppers and onion into small pieces. Place all ingredients in a cooking pan and simmer for 25 minutes.

Nutritional Instructions

Calories: 366 kcal, Fat: 9g, Carbs: 22g, Protein: 28g, Sugars: 0g, Fiber:10g

Pumpkin Soup

Serving size: 1

<u>Ingredients</u>

- 1 Ginger root
- 2 cups chopped Pumpkin
- 2 cups low-sodium vegetable broth
- 1 tbsp. Coconut Oil
- ¼ Onion
- 1 clove of Garlic

<u>Directions</u>

In a non-stick cooking pan, fry onion and garlic. Add onion and garlic to a pot with all other ingredients and boil for 20 minutes. Blend for a creamy texture.

<u>Nutritional Information</u>

Calories: 439 kcal, Fat: 27g, Carbs: 39g, Protein: 23g, Sugars: 0g, Fiber: 16g

Quinoa Bowl with Salmon

Serving size: 1

Ingredients

- ¼ cup quinoa
- 1pc. Salmon
- 1 cup vegetable broth
- ½ avocado
- 1 tbsp. olive oil
- Sesame seeds

Directions

Preheat the oven to 400°F/204°C. Drizzle olive oil onto the salmon and bake for 15 minutes. At the same time, add quinoa and vegetable broth into a pot and boil until cooked. Place cooked quinoa onto a plate with salmon and avocado. Top with sesame seeds.

Nutritional Information

Calories: 435 kcal, Fat: 19g, Carbs: 29g, Protein: 24g, Sugars: 2g, Fiber: 11g

Beef Power Bowl

Serving size: 1

<u>Ingredients</u>

- 3 oz beef
- ⅓ cup basmati rice
- ¼ cup cilantro
- ¼ cucumber
- ½ cup shredded carrots
- ½ cup green onion
- 1 tbsp. olive oil
- ¼ tsp. garlic powder
- Parsley
- 2 tbsp. soy sauce
- Handful of peanuts (optional)

<u>Directions</u>

Boil 1 cup of water in a pot, add the rice, and let it simmer on low temperature for 12 minutes. Cut beef into pieces. On a non-stick cooking pan add oil and cook the garlic and beef for 5 minutes, stirring often. Add cooked rice and beef to a bowl, then add carrots, cucumber, green onion, and parsley on top. Drizzle on soy sauce. Add peanuts for extra flavor.

Nutritional Information

Calories: 385 kcal, Fat: 23g, Carbs: 29g, Protein: 26g, Sugars: 1g, Fiber: 12g

Three Bean Soup

Serving size: 1

Ingredients

- ¼ cup kidney beans
- ¼ cup pinto beans
- ¼ cup chickpeas
- 2 tbsp. corn
- 1 tomato
- 2 cups low-sodium vegetable broth
- Black pepper
- ½ chili pepper
- 1 tbsp. Olive oil

Directions

Place all of the ingredients in a cooking pot and boil for 30 minutes. Serve and top with parsley if desired.

Nutritional Information

Calories: 458 kcal, Fat: 23g, Carbs: 35g, Protein: 26g, Sugars: 1g, Fiber: 12g

Pesto Shrimp Risotto

Serving size: 1

<u>Ingredients</u>

- 1 cup fresh shrimp
- ½ cup basmati rice
- 1 cup vegetable broth
- 2 tbsp. pesto
- ½ cup green beans
- 1 tbs. olive oil
- Salt
- Pepper

<u>Directions</u>

Spread 1 tsp. olive oil in a cooking pan, and sauté the shrimp and green beans for 10 minutes, turning the shrimp over after 5 minutes. Boil vegetable broth and add in the rice, simmer for 10 minutes. Stir in pesto, salt, and pepper and simmer for another 5 minutes. Place cooked rice on a plate with shrimp.

<u>Nutritional Information</u>

Calories: 456 kcal, Fat: 25g, Carbs: 29g, Protein: 32g, Sugars: 2g, Fiber: 3g

Now that you know how to make all those delicious recipes, let's put it all together! Follow my weight loss meal plan below to ensure no one suspects that you've joined the Menopause Weight Distribution Club!

Day 1

Breakfast: Almond Flour Pancakes

Lunch: Quinoa Bowl

Dinner: Chicken Stir Fry

Day 2

Breakfast: Egg Muffin Bites

Lunch: Stuffed Pepper

Dinner: Salmon and Noodles

Day 3

Breakfast: Blueberry Oatmeal Bowl

Lunch: Salmon and Spinach Salad

Dinner: Taco Bowl

Day 4

Breakfast: Avocado Toast with Poached Eggs

Lunch: Zucchini Pasta with Ground Beef

Dinner: Chicken Fajitas

Day 5

Breakfast: Anti-Inflammatory Smoothie

Lunch: Mediterranean Veggie Wrap

Dinner: Shrimp Dish with Veggies

Day 6

Breakfast: Yogurt Fruit Bowl

Lunch: Falafel Avocado Wrap with Garlic Aioli

Dinner: Ground Turkey Chili

Day 7

Breakfast: Apple Muffins

Lunch: Chicken Salad

Dinner: Quinoa Bowl with Salmon

Day 8

Breakfast: Detox Protein Smoothie

Lunch: Chicken Protein Soup

Dinner: Pesto Shrimp Risotto

Day 9

Breakfast: Overnight Kiwi and Chia

Lunch: Chicken Teriyaki and Salad

Dinner: Chickpea Stew

Day 10

Breakfast: Spinach Omelet

Lunch: Tabouli Salad

Dinner: Beef Power Bowl

Day 11

Breakfast: Yogurt Banana Split

Lunch: Chicken and Veggie Skewers

Dinner: Pumpkin Soup

Day 12

Breakfast: Pineapple Kale Smoothie

Lunch: Stuffed Pepper

Dinner: Chicken Stir Fry

Day 13

Breakfast: Egg Muffin Bites

Lunch: Spinach Frittata With Millet

Dinner: Pesto Shrimp Risotto

Day 14

Breakfast: Anti-Inflammatory Smoothie

Lunch: Quinoa Bowl

Dinner: Chicken Stir Fry

Day 15

Breakfast: Almond Flour Pancakes

Lunch: Chicken Salad

Dinner: Three Bean Soup

Day 16

Breakfast: Spinach Omelet

Lunch: Falafel Avocado Wrap with Garlic Aioli

Dinner: Salmon and Noodles

Day 17

Breakfast: Blueberry Oatmeal Bowl

Lunch: Chicken Teriyaki and Salad

Dinner: Taco Bowl

Day 18

Breakfast: Apple Muffins

Lunch: Salmon and Spinach Salad

Dinner: Chickpea Stew

Day 19

Breakfast: Avocado Toast with Poached Eggs

Lunch: Quinoa Bowl

Dinner: Chicken Fajitas

Day 20

Breakfast: Anti-Inflammatory Smoothie

Lunch: Mediterranean Veggie Wrap

Dinner: Ground Turkey Chili

Day 21

Breakfast: Yogurt Fruit Bowl

Lunch: Chicken Protein Soup

Dinner: Beef Power Bowl

Day 22

Breakfast: Detox Protein Smoothie

Lunch: Stuffed Pepper

Dinner: Quinoa Bowl with Salmon

Day 23

Breakfast: Overnight Kiwi and Chia

Lunch: Tabouli Salad

Dinner: Shrimp Dish with Veggies

Day 24

Breakfast: Egg Muffin Bites

Lunch: Zucchini Pasta with Ground Beef

Dinner: Pumpkin Soup

Day 25

Breakfast: Pineapple Kale Smoothie

Lunch: Spinach Frittata With Millet

Dinner: Salmon and Noodles

Day 26

Breakfast: Spinach Omelet

Lunch: Chicken and Veggie Skewers

Dinner: Chickpea Stew

Day 27

Breakfast: Yogurt Banana Split

Lunch: Spinach Frittata With Millet

Dinner: Pesto Shrimp Risotto

Day 28

Breakfast: Blueberry Oatmeal Bowl

Lunch: Chicken Protein Soup

Dinner: Beef Power Bowl

As we bid farewell to this chapter, remember that healthy eating can be like learning to ride a unicycle, awkward at first but guaranteed to turn heads. As we move on, let's explore some other ways to look and feel like the best version of yourself during menopause!

8

HOW TO LOOK HOT AND FEEL FABULOUS

E veryone wants to look beautiful. Sure, we're not all going to achieve that "I can afford all the plastic surgery in the world" look, but we can still look dashing enough to turn heads (and maybe cause a few traffic accidents).

"Your honor, the defendant is accused of causing a ten-car pile-up by looking too damn sexy! Hence, the prosecutor believes the defendant should be locked up until a time when she stops being a stone-cold fox, posing a risk to all of us and to our safety."

By following my 28-day meal plan and a good exercise routine, you're well on your way to looking like a stone-cold fox. The final step is your hair, skin, lips, and nails.

In this chapter, we will focus on the effects of menopause on your hair, skin, lips, and nail health, and I will provide tips and supplements to manage any not-so-pleasant symptoms of these important beauty parts so that you look and feel hot.

MENOPAUSE VS. YOUR SKIN

During menopause, your skin and hair are like two wilting plants in the scorching sun. They are drying out, losing their color, and begging for water. Fortunately, you can water the plants (skin and hair) back to life with supplements and self-care tips. Let's start with your skin.

In the previous chapter, we talked about collagen and how that bad boy keeps our skin looking supple, youthful, and tender. According to the American Academy of Dermatology Association, "In menopause, skin quickly loses collagen. Studies show that women's skin loses about 30% of its collagen during the first five years of menopause. After that, the decline is more gradual. Women lose about 2% of their collagen every year for the next 20 years. As collagen diminishes, our skin loses its firmness and begins to sag. Jowls appear." Before you panic, there is hope for slowing down this aging process and still looking like a regal queen. Keep reading and you will get to the gold treasure soon!

Estrogen also keeps our skin well-hydrated. A well-hydrated skin is a plump, juicy skin. Unfortunately, with lower estrogen levels, you lose all this juicy hydration and begin to notice other symptoms like:

- Skin sagging
- Loss of skin volume
- Skin dryness or flaking
- Age spots
- Postmenopausal acne

Additionally, you may notice unwanted hair growth on your upper lip and chin thanks to the ever-generous hormonal changes.

Caring for your Skin in Menopause

To care for your skin in menopause:

- Always apply sunscreen

Ask any skincare expert what the secret to good skin is, and this is the number one advice they give to prevent a whole bunch of skin problems. The sun is no joke, and our puny human skin is just no match for it! Always apply sunscreen.

- Attend regular skin cancer screenings

Your risk of skin cancer increases as you age. Ask your dermatologist to teach you how to do regular skin self-exams to look for signs of cancer in between appointments. Your dermatologist will also be able to help you safely remove unwanted facial hair and help you if you have any problems with acne.

(Always make sure your dermatologist is board-certified.)

- Swap from soaps to mild cleansers

Soaps are often harsh and dry on the skin, unlike mild cleansers.

- Moisturize!

What makes a freshly roasted turkey look so juicy and enticing? You basted it with oils! The same principle applies to your skin. Baste yourself like a turkey and moisturize!

In the past, people simply stayed out all day in the sun, washed their faces with any soap they could find, and never moisturized. That's why they had wrinkles by the time they turned twenty, a deep tan that no amount of acid or laser treatments in this world would remove, and skin cancer by the time they turned thirty. As we learn more about the importance of skincare, we're all now taking better care of our skin - and looking gorgeous as a result!

Lastly, ask your dermatologist about using tretinoin (or any other alternatives, such as gentler retinol or peptides). Apart from sunscreen, tretinoin is the second most important skincare product for keeping your skin freshly-basted!

MENOPAUSE VS. YOUR HAIR

For some women, the first symptoms of peri-menopause or menopause that they notice are changes in their hair, like having to unclog the drain in the bathroom more often or seeing large clumps of your hair on the floor after brushing, like you would see at the hairdressers. It's sort of an understatement to say that this can be really shocking, particularly if you've always been able to boast of healthy, luxurious hair before. You used to be unable to run your fingers through your hair because it was so full and thick, and now it seems your hair is thinning by the day, falling out at concerning speed and breaking just for the hell of it. Some women even notice thinning patches on their scalp and even pubic regions. On the plus side, another possible change is a lack of hair growth on your legs, arms, and armpit, so you do get to save on shaving sticks and wax appointments.

These are all common symptoms of menopause that occur because your estrogen and progesterone levels are not at the level they used to be pre-menopause. With declining levels of these two hormones, your body switches to producing more androgens. Androgens are typically produced at higher levels in men and are a big reason why balding is a common issue men face as opposed to women. One side effect of increased androgen production in the body is causing the hair follicles on your body to shrink, leading to hair loss. It is also possible for some medications that women over 40 are prescribed to cause hair loss, such as antidepressants, heart medications, and medications to treat hyperthyroidism. On the other hand, medications prescribed to treat symptoms of menopause actually tend to improve your hair, so if you are on any medication that is not related to menopause, speak with your doctor to determine if it is the cause of changes in your hair.

Caring for your Hair at Menopause

• Rogaine (minoxidil)

So, scientists can take us to the moon but still can't figure out a pill to reverse hair loss without any other side effects? As if any astronaut wants to travel through space and meet aliens without a full head of shiny, luxurious hair.

Whoever develops this pill will definitely become an overnight billionaire, so why am I giving you the idea in the first place? Finally, something to do in my secret lab!

Until I can develop this pill, you can use Rogaine (minoxidil), which has been proven to treat hair loss. It does come with side effects, such as scalp dryness, flaking, itchiness, and even burning. Although rare, there are severe side effects too, like weight gain, light-headedness, chest pain, increased heartbeat, and swelling of the face.

• Eat protein-rich food.

Your hair is made out of a protein known as keratin. The more protein you eat, the more keratin is available for your hair to stay strong and full.

• Use hair products with vitamin C

Also known as ascorbic acid, vitamin C helps remove mineral buildup in hair, improving your hair's ability to absorb moisture and stay healthy.

• Eat vitamin-A-rich foods

Vitamin A is necessary for increasing the speed of cell regeneration and synthesis, two processes that improve hair growth.

• Other vitamins and minerals great for your hair's health are:

- Iron
- Niacin
- Vitamin B12
- Pantothenic acid (vitamin B5)
- Healthy fats from sources like avocados, olive oil, nuts and seeds
- Zinc

You can also take supplements to ensure you are getting enough of these nutrients. Still, make sure to speak with your doctor first before you begin taking supplements, especially if you are currently on any medication.

• Use hair extensions

If the side effects of minoxidil don't seem particularly enticing, or if you can't be bothered to wait for the effects of your lifestyle changes to kick in, don't discount the use of extensions, weaves, and wigs. All your favorite celebrities wear them, yes, even the menopausal and postmenopausal ones. I have a client who runs her own hairdresser, and you would be shocked at how many women use some form of extensions to make their hair fuller or longer, or to change their hair color without damaging it. The use of wigs and hair transplant operations has also become a common practice among men, who are suspiciously bald one day and suddenly have a full head of shiny, wavy Arabian curls the next.

All this to say, everyone is doing it and lying about it, so don't feel ashamed to add a little bit of clip-ins here and there or to use a nice wig to your daughter's wedding so the pictures turn out alright. Just make sure to learn how to install them properly or get a recommended professional to do them for you to avoid wig-related embarrassments!

MENOPAUSE VS. YOUR NAILS

"Menopause. Estrogen. Collagen. Protein. Keratin. Moisture loss... Ella, we get it! Estrogen can affect your nails. Just skip to the part with steps for how to make my nails look good!" Fair enough.

Ways to Manage Brittle Nails

- Check for iron deficiencies

Iron deficiencies can cause brittle and dry nails. Your nails are made of the same keratin as your hair, so the same vitamins and minerals that cause healthy hair also lead to healthy nails. Hence, the more you take care of your hair, the more healthy your nails become.

- Moisturize!

Just like your skin and hair, your nails like being moisturized. Since we spend all day washing our hands, doing the dishes, cooking, etc., it is easy to leave your nails dry from too much water exposure. Always keep a small fancy tub of lotion nearby to moisturize. Plus, you'll look so fancy and classy opening it up and moisturizing your hands while the rest of the unclassy commoners don't even pay attention to their hands!

- Use a nail hardener

As well as a nail hardener, trim and file nails often to prevent splitting and breaking.

- Be patient

Nails take time to grow and get healthy again, just like skin and hair. Be patient and give it about six months. If you don't notice changes, then you can see a doctor to find out what is causing your unhealthy nails. Furthermore, regardless of menopause, our fingernails do grow thinner and more brittle (while our toenails grow thicker and harder) as we age, so a bit of acceptance goes a long way (as well as removing chemicals from your nail regime, such as acetone or nail gels).

If the steps above don't see a marked improvement in your nail health, you should also check with your doctor that your unhealthy nails are not a result of an underactive thyroid gland, Raynaud's syndrome, or a fungal infection.

MENOPAUSE VS. YOUR LIPS

We all need juicy lips. Yes, need. There is no argument here. We need it like we need oxygen or food! I will be taking no comments.

To reduce the amount of juiciness being siphoned from your lips during menopause:

- Eat anti-inflammatory foods

Inflammation further decreases collagen levels in our body, so you want to prevent inflammation as much as possible.

- Practice stress-relieving exercises

This will help to reduce inflammation further.

- Wear sunscreen

People don't realize that you can wear sunscreen on your lips, underneath any lip products you're wearing, but you can.

- Take collagen supplements

There is ongoing debate in the scientific community about whether hydrolyzed collagen peptides work, but I take them and notice my hair and lips grow fuller when I do.

- Stop smoking

Besides preventing you from dying, one other equally important reason to stop smoking is to prevent your lips from thinning out.

- Drink water

Besides also stopping you from dying, water's other primary function is to keep your lips full. Oh, and I guess other lesser important functions like keeping your organs healthy, but who *really* needs that?

- Invest in a good lip treatment

They are loaded with great ingredients to improve your lips from the outside in.

- Kiss more

OK, I added this on my own with no scientific proof whatsoever. However, I figured kissing leads to sex, and sex leads to relaxation and happiness, and happiness and relaxation leads to less inflammation, and less inflammation leads to plumper lips, hence kissing is directly related to plump lips. Now, *that's* science.

Don't forget another important aspect of looking hot: the way you dress. No one is saying you should wear booty shorts and stripper heels to your granddaughter's christening. However, you can still dress to look good by emphasizing your best features and body parts.

Plus, menopause does not mean you can't wear booty shorts. It simply means you have to carefully choose the appropriate time to wear them, like on your way to buy organic produce at the farmer's market. Or on your wedding day, to let your spouse know that, with a butt this gorgeous, they can be replaced at any time!

CONCLUSION

Menopause is a beautiful season in your life. Don't let anyone tell you differently. As Davina McCall said, it used to mean the sunset of life for most women back in the days when advances in modern science and medicine had not increased our life expectancy. Today, women are spending one-third to one-half of their lives postmenopause. How then can life possibly be over after living just half of it? It's absolutely ridiculous! Sure, at first glance, it feels as though menopause brings nothing but headache and pain, but that's before you learned of all the treatment options available to slow down the process, alleviate your symptoms, improve your life, wear booty shorts, have kegel sex, and essentially flip menopause the proverbial bird.

In this book, I have given you the essential guide for looking menopause in the eye and asserting dominance! Using scientifically-proven methods and treatments, such as hormone therapy, exercise, diet, and supplements, you can live the second part of your life with the full vigor and vivaciousness as you did your first half, haters be damned! You are now fully empowered with all the different symptoms of menopause and how to treat them. You know how to deal with depression, insomnia, anxiety, and hot flashes and still walk out there, ready to be arrested for being just too damn fine for the safety of your community! You may not have a hidden secret beauty well, but you have the next best thing: knowledge. And, if knowledge is power, then that makes you the strongest menopausal woman in the world.

Now that you know how to treat your symptoms, the next step is to go out there and enjoy the new world you've been reborn into! After thirty or more years, you no longer have to carry an extra tampon with you, have to deal with periods and the ups and downs of a menstrual cycle, or the absolute gut-wrenching fear that comes from a missed or late period. You can have spine-tingling sex without worrying about accidentally getting pregnant. Without caring what people think anymore, you can finally dye your hair the color you always wanted. If anyone doesn't approve, let's see if they have the audacity to face you in your newly empowered form!

As if the positives aren't enough, you can now learn a new sexuality that is based on confidence, knowing who you are, and knowing that, despite all you went through, you're still standing strong. You can begin to speak up and advocate for other women who are about to go through menopause too, keeping in mind that, until the world begins to take menopausal women seriously, we won't rest! They're just going to have to arrest you for being both too damn fine and too damn powerful!

Now that you're equipped with all the information you need to start your journey to losing weight and looking hot after menopause, don't keep it all to yourself! Women need to know how to stop traffic and still feel great despite estrogen betraying us! Perhaps if enough of us begin to stop traffic with our jaw-dropping gorgeousness, governments and scientists worldwide will begin to take notice and be forced to take menopause more seriously! In the meantime, leave a review, so we can begin the menopausal revolution!

MY BOOKS

Simple Methods For Women's Gut Health That Work

Tips and Tricks to Improve Digestion, Restore Your Health & Recharge Your Body and Mind

Conquer Emotional Eating

Overcome Negative Thoughts and Self-Sabotage. Take Control of Your Body and Your Life Today.

The 5 Step Hormone Secret To Weight Loss For Women

The Little-Known Solution to Resetting Your Adrenal Glands, Boosting Your Metabolism, Elevating Your Mood, and Losing Weight Once and for All

REFERENCES

"10 Nutrients for Healthy Hair During Menopause - Marion Gluck." n.d. The Marion Gluck Clinic. Accessed July 7, 2023. https://www.mariongluckclinic.com/blog/nutrients-healthy-hair-menopause.html.

"10 Tips for a Healthy Diet After Age 50." 2023. AgingCare. Accessed July 6, 2023. https://www.agingcare.com/articles/nutrition-tips-for-elderly-health-and-diets-137 053.htm.

Ajmera, Rachel, and Kiara Anthony. 2021. "Adrenal Fatigue Diet: Good and Bad Foods for Adrenal Health." Healthline. https://www.health line.com/health/adrenal-fatigue-diet#foods-to-avoid.

Asamoah, Tracy, and Jillian Amodio. 2021. "How Menopause Affects Your Mental Health." GoodRx. https://www.goodrx.com/conditions/menopause/how-menopause-affects-your-men tal-health.

"As Menopause Nears, Be Aware It Can Trigger Depression and Anxiety, Too." 2023.

NPR.org. https://www.npr.org/sections/health-shots/2020/01/16/796682276/for-some-wom en-nearing-menopause-depression-and-anxiety-can-spike.

Barraclough, A. (2022). "10 celebrities who've openly shared their menopause experiences", helping the condition to become mainstream. *Marie Claire UK*. https://www.marieclaire.co.uk/life/health-fitness/celebrities-menopause-797175

Bhanote, Monisha. 2022. "7 of the best essential oils for sleep." Medical News Today. https://www.medicalnewstoday.com/articles/essen tial-oils-for-sleep#pros-and-cons

Babakhanian, Masoudeh, Masumeh Ghazanfarpour, Leila Kargarfard, Nasibeh Roozbeh, Leili Darvish, Talat Khadivzadeh, and Fatemeh Rajab Dizavandi. 2018. "Effect of Aromatherapy on the Treatment of Psychological Symptoms in Postmenopausal and Elderly Women: A Systematic Review and Meta-Analysis." Journal of

Menopausal Medicine 24 (2): 127. https://doi.org/10.6118/jmm. 2018.24.2.127.

Barraclough, Alice. 2022. "10 celebrities who've openly shared their menopause experiences, helping the condition to become mainstream." Marie Claire UK. https://www.marieclaire.co.uk/life/health-fitness/celebrities-menopause-797175.

Begum, Jabeen. 2023. "Menopause Emotions, Depression, Moodiness, and More." WebMD. https://www.webmd.com/menopause/emotional-roller-coaster.

Bottaro, Angelica. 2022. "Menopause and Hair Loss: Symptoms. Causes, and Treatment." Verywell Health. https://www.verywellhealth.com/menopause-hair-loss-5218350.

Brazier, Yvette. 2015. "Exercise eases hot flashes during menopause." Medical News Today. https://www.medicalnewstoday.com/articles/304295.

British Menopause Society. 2022. "Cognitive Behaviour Therapy (CBT) for Menopausal Symptoms." Women's Health Concern. https://www.womens-health-concern.org/wp-content/uploads/2023/02/02-WHCFACTSHEET-CBT-WOMEN-FEB-2023-A.pdf.

"Bruising during Menopause." 2019. Menopause Now. https://www.menopausenow.com/bruising-during-menopause.

"Caring for your skin in menopause." n.d. American Academy of Dermatology. Accessed July 7, 2023. https://www.aad.org/public/everyday-care/skin-care-secrets/anti-aging/skin-care-d uring-menopause.

CDC. 2018. "Products - Data Briefs - Number 313 - July 2018." Centers for Disease Control and Prevention. https://www.cdc.gov/nchs/products/databriefs/db313.htm.

Chalker, Rebecca. 2009. "Strategies for Staying Sexual After Menopause." National Women's Health Network. https://nwhn.org/strategies-for-staying-sexual-after-menopause/.

Cleveland Clinic. 2022. "Hormonal Imbalance: Causes, Symptoms & Treatment." Cleveland Clinic. April 4, 2022. https://my.clevelandclinic.org/health/diseases/22673-hormonal-imbalance.

Cleveland Clinic. 2021. "Hormone Therapy for Menopause: Types, Benefits & Risks." Cleveland Clinic. June 28, 2021. https://my.cleve-landclinic.org/health/treatments/15245-hormone-therapy-for-men opause-symptoms.

Cleveland Clinic. 2022. "Estrogen: Hormone, Function, Levels & Imbalances." Cleveland Clinic. August 2, 2022. https://my.cleveland clinic.org/health/body/22353-estrogen.

Conde, Délio Marques, Roberto Carmignani Verdade, Ana L R Valadares, Lucas F B

Mella, Adriana Orcesi Pedro, and Lucia Costa-Paiva. 2021. "Menopause and Cognitive Impairment: A Narrative Review of Current Knowledge." *World Journal of Psychiatry* 11 (8): 412–28. https://doi.org/10.5498/wjp.v11.i8.412.

Davidson, M., and Kara L. Smythe. 2023. "9 Ways to Even Out Menopause Mood Swings - Menopause Center." Everyday Health. https://www.everydayhealth.com/menopause-pictures/ways-to-even-out-menopaus e-mood-swings.aspx.

"Does menopause affect your ears?" 2021. A.Vogel. https://www.avo-gel.co.uk/health/menopause/videos/does-menopause-affect-your-e ars/.

Durward, Eileen. 2021. "Does menopause affect your ears?" A.Vogel. https://www.avogel.co.uk/health/menopause/videos/does-menopause-affect-your-e ars/.

Eagleson, Claire, Sarra Hayes, Andrew Mathews, Gemma Perman, and Colette R. Hirsch. 2016. "The Power of Positive Thinking: Pathological Worry Is Reduced by Thought Replacement in Generalized Anxiety Disorder." *Behaviour Research and Therapy* 78 (78): 13–18. https://doi.org/10.1016/j.brat.2015.12.017.

"Effects of Menopause on the Body." 2019. Healthline. February 5, 2019. https://www.healthline.com/health/menopause/hrt-effects-on-body#Cardiovascula r-system.

Engler, Alexandra. 2020. "Lips Thin With Age: Why It Happens + What To Do About It | mindbodygreen." MindBodyGreen. https://www.mindbodygreen.com/articles/lips-thin-with-age.

Ernst, Holly, and Noreen Iftikhar. 2018. "Antidepressants for

Menopause: Benefits, Types, Side Effects, and More." Healthline. https://www.healthline.com/health/antidepressants-for-menopause#side-effects.

Everly Well. 2023. "Your Complete Guide to Sex After Menopause." Everlywell. https://www.everlywell.com/blog/womens-health/sex-after-menopause/.

FDA. Commissioner, Office of the. 2019. "Menopause: Medicines to Help You." *FDA*, September. https://www.fda.gov/consumers/free-publications-women/menopause-medicines-h elp-you.

Fletcher, J. (2023, January 5). *How long do menopause symptoms last?* https://www.medicalnewstoday.com/articles/314951

Forth. 2020. "Menopause Hormones - What Are They and How Do They Change?" Forth. October 28, 2020. https://www.forthwith life.co.uk/blog/menopause-hormones/.

Fry, Alexa, and Alex Dimitriu. 2023. "Stress and Insomnia." Sleep Foundation. https://www.sleepfoundation.org/insomnia/stress-and-insomnia.

Garrard, C. (2023, April 7). *"Coping with hot flashes and other menopausal symptoms: What 16 celebrities said".* EverydayHealth.com. https://www.everydayhealth.com/menopause/coping-hot-flashes-menopausal-symptoms-celebrities-said/

Gaudon, Ann M. 2018. "The Link Between Trauma and Chronic Pain — Pain News Network." Pain News Network. https://www.-painnewsnetwork.org/stories/2018/5/25/the-link-between-trauma-an d-chronic-pain.

Gee, Madelyn, Anthony Rivas, and Alicia Valenski. 2022. "How Exercise Releases 'Feel-Good' Hormones." Www.theskimm.com. March 11, 2022. https://www.theskimm.com/wellness/hormones-released-during-exercise-endorphi ns.

Guidi, Mark. 2016. "5 Scientific Studies that Prove the Power of Positive Thinking." LinkedIn. https://www.linkedin.com/pulse/5-scientific-studies-prove-power-positive-thinking -mark-guidi.

"Healthy Eating and Diet Tips for Women." 2023. HelpGuide.org. https://www.helpguide.org/articles/healthy-eating/diet-and-nutri-tion-tips-for-wom en.htm.

Heart of Florida OB/GYN. (2020). "What are the most common myths and misconceptions about menopause?" *Advanced OB/GYN*. https://advancedobgynlakecounty.com/what-are-the-most-common-myths-and-misconceptions-about-menopause/

"Hormone Replacement Therapy: What to Know." 2023. Verywell Health. https://www.verywellhealth.com/hormone-replacement-therapy-5271199.

"Hormones 101: Meet 7 Important Hormones." 2022. Cleveland Clinic. July 19, 2022. https://health.clevelandclinic.org/what-are-hormones/.

"Hot Flashes: Triggers, How Long They Last & Treatments." n.d. Cleveland Clinic. https://my.clevelandclinic.org/health/articles/15223-hot-flashes.

"Hot Flashes: What Can I Do? | National Institute on Aging." 2023. National Institute on Aging. https://www.nia.nih.gov/health/hot-flashes-what-can-i-do.

"How Can Exercise Affect Sleep?" 2023. Sleep Foundation. https://www.sleepfoundation.org/physical-activity/exercise-and-sleep.

"How Can Menopause Affect Sleep?" 2022. Sleep Foundation. https://www.sleepfoundation.org/women-sleep/menopause-and-sleep.

"How Does Menopause Affect Your Appearance." 2023. Solace Women's Care. https://www.solacewomenscare.com/blog/how-does-menopause-affect-your-appear ance.

"How Hormone Depletion Affects You | Menopause." 2023. Menopause.obgyn.msu.edu. https://menopause.obgyn.msu.edu/content/how-hormone-depletion-affects-you.

"How Menopause Affects Your Mental Health | Let's Talk Menopause." 2023. Www.letstalkmenopause.org. https://www.letstalk menopause.org/menopause-mental-health.

"How menopause can affect your heart." 2020. Edward-Elmhurst Health. https://www.eehealth.org/blog/2020/07/how-menopause-can-affect-your-heart/.

"How to Increase Estrogen with These 11 Power Foods." 2019. Healthline. August 23, 2019. https://www.healthline.com/nutri tion/foods-with-estrogen#TOC_TITLE_HDR_10.

Hi, Su, and Freeman Ew. 2009. "Hormone Changes Associated with the Menopausal Transition.," Minerva Ginecol, 61(6): 483–489.

Iavarone, K. (2022). Do menopause home tests work? 5 options to consider. *www.medicalnewstoday.com*. https://www.medicalnewsto day.com/articles/menopause-home-tests

ITV. 2020. "Davina McCall on menopause: 'I was waking up soaked in sweat thinking there was something wrong with me.'" ITVX. https://www.itv.com/loosewomen/articles/davina-mccall-opens-up-about-menopau se.

Joly, Louise. 2011. "Exercise, Nature and Socially Interactive Based Initiatives Improve Mood and Self-Esteem in the Clinical Population." *Primary Health Care* 21 (7): 15–15. https://doi.org/10.7748/phc.21.7.15.s9.

Jones, Brandi. 2022. "Menopause and Heart Palpitations." Verywell Health. https://www.verywellhealth.com/menopause-and-heart-palpitations-5218109.

Joshi, Sulabha, and Nirmala Vaze. 2010. "Yoga and Menopausal Transition." *Journal of Mid-Life Health* 1 (2): 56. https://doi.org/10.4103/0976-7800.76212.

Klein, Alex. 2020. "How to stop a panic attack: 13 effective methods." Medical News Today. https://www.medicalnewstoday.com/arti cles/321510#methods.

Kubala, Kendra. 2021. "Menopause and insomnia: Link, duration, and remedies." Medical News Today. https://www.medicalnewstoday.-com/articles/menopause-and-insomnia#compleme ntary-therapies.

LaMantia, B., & Ma, J. (2022, February 15). 25 "Famous women on getting older". *The Cut*. https://www.thecut.com/article/25-famous-women-on-aging.html

Lee, Youngwhee, and Hwasoon Kim. 2008. "Relationships between Menopausal Symptoms, Depression, and Exercise in Middle-Aged Women: A Cross-Sectional Survey." *International Journal of Nursing Studies* 45 (12): 1816–22. https://doi.org/10.1016/j.ijnurstu.2008.07.001.

Lovell, Rachel. 2023. "Why modern food lost its nutrients." BBC.

https://www.bbc.com/future/bespoke/follow-the-food/why-modern-food-lost-its-n utrients/.

"Low Testosterone in Women: Signs, Causes, and Treatments." 2018. Www.medicalnewstoday.com. August 2, 2018. https://www. medicalnewstoday.com/articles/322663#causes.

MacMillan, C. 2018. Women, How Good Are Your Eggs? Yale Medicine. https://www.yalemedicine.org/news/fertility-test.

Mayo Clinic. 2023. "Headaches and hormones: What's the connection?" Mayo Clinic. https://www.mayoclinic.org/diseases-conditions/chronic-daily-headaches/in-depth /headaches/art-20046729.

Mead, Liz. 2021. "Menopause and Dry Eyes: Is There a Connection?" Bonafide. https://hellobonafide.com/blogs/news/dry-eyes-and-menopause.

"Menopause" | Office on Women's Health. (n.d.). https://www.women shealth.gov/menopause

"Menopause - Diagnosis and treatment" - Mayo Clinic. (2023, May 25). https://www.mayoclinic.org/diseases-conditions/menopause/diag nosis-treatment/drc-20353401

"Menopause and Fibromyalgia." 2023. Fibromyalgia Symptoms. Accessed July 6, 2023. https://www.fibromyalgia-symptoms.org/menopause-fibromyalgia.html.

"Menopause and Melatonin | University of Utah Health." 2021. University of Utah Health. https://healthcare.utah.edu/the-scope/health-library/all/2021/05/menopause-andmelatonin.

"Menopause: the different stages". (n.d.). Apollo247. https://www.apol lo247.com/blog/article/menopause-different-stages

"Menopause - Symptoms and causes" - Mayo Clinic. (2023, May 25). Mayo Clinic. https://www.mayoclinic.org/diseases-conditions/menopause/symptoms-causes/syc-20353397

"Menopause Weight Loss - How Exercise Can Help! - Blog - HealthifyMe." 2022. Healthifyme. https://www.healthifyme.com/blog/lose-weight-with-exercise-during-menopause/.

Nast, Condé. 2020. "10 Celebrities Who Have Spoken out about

Menopause." Glamour. October 5, 2020. https://www.glamour.-com/gallery/celebrities-who-have-spoken-out-about-menopa use.

Newsom, Rob, and Alex Dimitriu. 2023. "Depression and Sleep." Sleep Foundation. https://www.sleepfoundation.org/mental-health/depression-and-sleep.

Obesity Action Coalition. (2021, August 5). *"The Truth about Menopause and Weight Gain" - Obesity Action Coalition.* https://www.obesityaction.org/resources/the-truth-about-menopause-and-weight-gain/

Paul. (2017). "7 common misconceptions about Menopause". *Balance Hormone Center.* https://www.balancehormonecenter.com/blog/7-common-misconceptions-menopause/

Payne, Jennifer. n.d. "Can Menopause Cause Depression?" Johns Hopkins Medicine. Accessed June 23, 2023. https://www.hopkinsmedicine.org/health/wellness-and-prevention/can-menopause - cause-depression.

Professional, C. C. M. (n.d.). « »*Menopause".* Cleveland Clinic. https://my.clevelandclinic.org/health/diseases/21841-menopause

"Progesterone for Menopause Symptoms: Benefits and Side Effects." 2020. Healthline. September 18, 2020. https://www.healthline.-com/health/progesterone-for-menopause#hormone-replace ment.

Rotter, J. (2019, March 8). *"Menopause: 11 things Every Woman should know".* Healthline. https://www.healthline.com/health/menopause/menopause-facts#weight-gain

Savage, Amanda. n.d. "Best Pelvic Floor Exercises to Do in Menopause." Stella. Accessed July 7, 2023. https://www.onstella.com/the-latest/pelvic-floor/best-pelvic-floor-exercises/.

Scaccia, A. (2023, June 30). *"How long do symptoms of menopause last?"* Healthline. https://www.healthline.com/health/menopause/how-long-does-menopause-last

Segerstrom, Suzanne C., and Gregory E. Miller. 2004. "Psychological Stress and the Human Immune System: A Meta-Analytic Study of 30 Years of Inquiry." *Psychological Bulletin* 130 (4): 601–30. https://doi.org/10.1037/0033-2909.130.4.601.

"Serotonin: What Is It, Function & Levels." 2022. Cleveland Clinic. https://my.clevelandclinic.org/health/articles/22572-serotonin.

Shaw, Gina. 2023. "Over 50? Get Tips for Losing Weight." WebMD. Accessed July 7, 2023. https://www.webmd.com/healthy-aging/features/losing-weight-after-fifty.

Spencer, Clare. 2021. "Menopause Symptoms | Changes to Nails." My Menopause Centre. https://www.mymenopausecentre.com/symptoms/changes-to-nails/.

Suni, E. and Singh, A. 2023. "How Much Sleep Do We Really Need?" Sleep Foundation. https://www.sleepfoundation.org/how-sleep-works/how-much-sleep-do-we-really-n eed.

"The Menopause Sleep Survival Guide: Staying Cool at Night." 2021. HercLéon. https://hercleon.com/blogs/herctalk/the-menopause-sleep-survival-guide-staying-c ool-at-night.

"The Power of Positive Thinking." 2023. Johns Hopkins Medicine. https://www.hopkinsmedicine.org/health/wellness-and-prevention/the-power-of-p ositive-thinking.

Tello, Monique. 2020. "Menopause and insomnia: Could a low-GI diet help?" Harvard Health. https://www.health.harvard.edu/blog/menopause-and-insomnia-could-a-low-gi-die t-help-2020011718710.

"The Best Exercises to Help You Lose Weight During Menopause." 2021. Evernow. https://www.evernow.com/learn/the-best-exercises-to-help-you-lose-weight-during -menopause.

UPMC. 2023. "Mental Health Concerns During the Perimenopause." UPMC. https://www.upmc.com/services/south-central-pa/women/services/behavioral-heal th/conditions/perimenopause.

UpToDate. 2023. Menopausal Hot Flashes. UpToDate. https://www.uptodate.com/contents/menopausal-hot-flashes

Vogel, K. (2023, February 14). "Whether you're 25 or 65, here are 50 menopause quotes that will resonate with every woman". *Parade: Entertainment, Recipes, Health, Life, Holidays.* https://parade.com/1239990/kaitlin-vogel/menopause-quotes/

Washington, Nicole. 2022. "Hormonal imbalance and depression: What to know." Medical News Today. https://www.medicalnewstoday.com/articles/hormonal-depression.

Watson, Stephanie. 2021. "Dopamine: The pathway to pleasure."

Harvard Health. https://www.health.harvard.edu/mind-and-mood/dopamine-the-pathway-to-pleasu re.

"What Are Hot Flashes? What Can You Do about Them?" 2023. WebMD. https://www.webmd.com/menopause/guide/menopause-hot-flashes.

"What Are The Stages Of Menopause?" (n.d.). https://www.gennev.com/education/stages-of-menopause

"What You Need to Know about Menopause." 2018. Healthline. January 17, 2018. https://www.healthline.com/health/menopause#home-remedies.

Wilson, Debra R., BC AHN, Corinne O'Keefe, and Ann M. Griff. 2017. "Menopause and Dry Eyes: Treatment and Causes." Healthline. https://www.healthline.com/health/menopause/menopause-and-dry-eyes#treatme nt.

"Working out boosts brain health." 2020. American Psychological Association. https://www.apa.org/topics/exercise-fitness/stress.

"Your guide to Menopause". (2002, February 5). WebMD. https://www.webmd.com/menopause/guide/menopause-information

"Yoga for Sleep." 2023. Johns Hopkins Medicine. https://www.hopkinsmedicine.org/health/wellness-and-prevention/yoga-for-sleep

www.ingramcontent.com/pod-product-compliance
Lightning Source LLC
Chambersburg PA
CBHW062127020426
42335CB00013B/1126